C. Martin
Detroit, MI
Feb 2000

IP
θ freq p³¹
node impurity $i(T)$
split function $\phi(S,T)$
tree cost $R(T)$ or tree quality
tree cost complexity $R_\alpha(T)$
complexity parameter α

×   survival analysis { outcome CA or all causes unclear no, don't match.

p. 94   p not defined
p. 97   hazar(d)
p. 130   x, y not defined
p. 141   'anything'?
p. 144   Zhang 1997 missing

? convolution p. 130.

Statistics for Biology and Health

Series Editors
K. Dietz, M. Gail, K. Krickeberg, B. Singer

Springer
New York
Berlin
Heidelberg
Barcelona
Hong Kong
London
Milan
Paris
Singapore
Tokyo

Statistics for Biology and Health

Klein/Moeschberger: Survival Analysis: Techniques for Censored and Truncated Data.
Kleinbaum: Logistic Regression: A Self-Learning Text.
Kleinbaum: Survival Analysis: A Self-Learning Text.
Lange: Mathematical and Statistical Methods for Genetic Analysis.
Manton/Singer/Suzman: Forecasting the Health of Elderly Populations.
Salsburg: The Use of Restricted Significance Tests in Clinical Trials.
Zhang/Singer: Recursive Partitioning in the Health Sciences.

Heping Zhang   Burton Singer

Recursive Partitioning in the Health Sciences

With 60 Illustrations

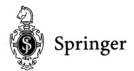
Springer

Heping Zhang
Department of Epidemiology
  and Public Health
School of Medicine
Yale University
60 College Street
New Haven, CT 06520-8034
USA

Burton Singer
Office of Population Research
Princeton University
Notestein Hall
21 Prospect Avenue
Princeton, NJ 08544
USA

Series Editors
K. Dietz
Institut für Medizinische Biometrie
Universität Tübingen
Westbahnhofstr. 55
D 72070 Tübingen
Germany

M. Gail
National Cancer Institute
Rockville, MD 20892
USA

K. Krickeberg
3 Rue de L'Estrapade
75005 Paris
France

B. Singer
Office of Population Research
Princeton University
Princeton, NJ 08544
USA

Library of Congress Cataloging-in-Publication Data
Zhang, Heping.
  Recursive partitioning in the health sceinces / Heping Zhang,
Burton Singer.
   p. cm. — (Statistics for biology and health)
  Includes bibliographical references and index.
  ISBN 0-387-98671-5 (alk. paper)
   1. Medicine—Research—Statistical methods. I. Singer, Burton.
II. Title. III. Series.
R853.S7 Z48 1999
610.7'27—ddc21   98-44699

Printed on acid-free paper.

© 1999 Springer-Verlag New York, Inc.
All rights reserved. This work may not be translated or copied in whole or in part without the written permission of the publisher (Springer-Verlag New York, Inc., 175 Fifth Avenue, New York, NY 10010, USA), except for brief excerpts in connection with reviews or scholarly analysis. Use in connection with any form of information storage and retrieval, electronic adaptation, computer software, or by similar or dissimilar methodology now known or hereafter developed is forbidden. The use of general descriptive names, trade names, trademarks, etc., in this publication, even if the former are not especially identified, is not to be taken as a sign that such names, as understood by the Trade Marks and Merchandise Marks Act, may accordingly be used freely by anyone.

Production managed by Timothy Taylor; manufacturing supervised by Jeffrey Taub.
Photocomposed copy prepared from the authors' LaTeX files.
Printed and bound by Edwards Brothers, Inc., Ann Arbor, MI.
Printed in the United States of America.

9 8 7 6 5 4 3 2 1

ISBN 0-387-98671-5 Springer-Verlag New York Berlin Heidelberg   SPIN 10699055

Dedicated to Julan, Jeffrey, and Leon

Preface

February 7, 2000

Multiple complex pathways, characterized by interrelated events and conditions, represent routes to many illnesses, diseases, and ultimately death. Although there are substantial data and plausibility arguments supporting many conditions as contributory components of pathways to illness and disease end points, we have, historically, lacked an effective methodology for identifying the structure of the full pathways. Regression methods, with strong linearity assumptions and data-based constraints on the extent and order of interaction terms, have traditionally been the strategies of choice for relating outcomes to potentially complex explanatory pathways. However, nonlinear relationships among candidate explanatory variables are a generic feature that must be dealt with in any characterization of how health outcomes come about. Thus, the purpose of this book is to demonstrate the effectiveness of a relatively recently developed methodology—recursive partitioning—as a response to this challenge. We also compare and contrast what is learned via recursive partitioning with results obtained on the same data sets using more traditional methods. This serves to highlight exactly where—and for what kinds of questions—recursive partitioning–based strategies have a decisive advantage over classical regression techniques.

This book is suitable for three broad groups of readers: (1) biomedical researchers, clinicians, public health practitioners including epidemiologists, health service researchers, environmental policy advisers; (2) consulting statisticians who can use the recursive partitioning technique as a guide in providing effective and insightful solutions to clients' problems; and (3) statisticians interested in methodological and theoretical issues. The book provides an up-to-date summary of the methodological and theoretical underpinnings of recursive partitioning. More interestingly, it presents a host of unsolved problems whose solutions would advance the rigorous underpinnings of statistics in general.

From the perspective of the first two groups of readers, we demonstrate with real applications the sequential interplay between automated production of multiple well-fitting trees and scientific judgment leading to respecification of variables, more refined trees subject to context-specific constraints (on splitting and pruning, for example), and ultimately selection of the most interpretable and useful tree(s). The sections marked with asterisks can be skipped for application-oriented readers.

We show a more conventional regression analysis—having the same objective as the recursive partitioning analysis—side by side with the newer methodology. In each example, we highlight the scientific insight derived from the recursive partitioning strategy that is not readily revealed by more conventional methods. The interfacing of automated output and scientific judgment is illustrated with both conventional and recursive partitioning analysis.

Theoretically oriented statisticians will find a substantial listing of challenging theoretical problems whose solutions would provide much deeper insight than heretofore about the scope and limits of recursive partitioning as such and multivariate adaptive splines in particular.

We emphasize the development of narratives to summarize the formal Boolean statements that define routes down the trees to terminal nodes. Particularly with complex—by scientific necessity—trees, narrative output facilitates understanding and interpretation of what has been provided by automated techniques.

We illustrate the sensitivity of trees to variation in choosing misclassification cost, where the variation is a consequence of divergent views by clinicians of the costs associated with differing mistakes in prognosis.

The book of Breiman et al. (1984) is a classical work on the subject of recursive partitioning. In Chapter 4, we reiterate the key ideas expressed in that book and expand our discussions in different directions on the issues that arise from applications. Other chapters on survival trees, adaptive splines, and classification trees for multiple discrete outcomes are new developments since the work of Breiman et al.

Heping Zhang wishes to thank his colleagues and students, Joan Buenconsejo, Theodore Holford, James Leckman, Ju Li, Robert Makuch, Kathleen Merikangas, Bradley Peterson, Norman Silliker, Daniel Zelterman, and Hongyu Zhao among others, for their help with reading and commenting on earlier drafts of this book. He is also grateful to Drs. Michael Bracken, Dorit Carmelli, and Brian Leaderer for making their data sets available to this book. This work was supported in part by NIH grant HD30712 to Heping Zhang.

Contents

Preface   vii

1 Introduction   1
   1.1 Examples Using CART 2
   1.2 The Statistical Problem 4
   1.3 Outline of the Methodology 5

2 A Practical Guide to Tree Construction   7
   2.1 The Elements of Tree Construction 9
   2.2 Splitting a Node 10
   2.3 Terminal Nodes 15
   2.4 Download and Use of Software 16

3 Logistic Regression   21
   3.1 Logistic Regression Models 21
   3.2 A Logistic Regression Analysis 22

4 Classification Trees for a Binary Response   29
   4.1 Node Impurity 29
   4.2 Determination of Terminal Nodes 32
      4.2.1 Misclassification Cost 32
      4.2.2 Cost Complexity 35
      4.2.3 Nested Optimal Subtrees* 37
   4.3 The Standard Error of R^{cv*} 40

	4.4	Tree-Based Analysis of the Yale Pregnancy Outcome Study	41
	4.5	An Alternative Pruning Approach	43
	4.6	Localized Cross-Validation	47
	4.7	Comparison Between Tree-Based and Logistic Regression Analyses	49
	4.8	Missing Data	53
		4.8.1 Missings Together Approach	53
		4.8.2 Surrogate Splits	54
	4.9	Tree Stability	55
	4.10	Implementation*	56

5 Risk-Factor Analysis Using Tree-Based Stratification   61
     5.1 Background   61
     5.2 The Analysis   63

6 Analysis of Censored Data: Examples   71
     6.1 Introduction   71
     6.2 Tree-Based Analysis for the Western Collaborative Group Study Data   74

7 Analysis of Censored Data: Concepts and Classical Methods   79
     7.1 The Basics of Survival Analysis   79
         7.1.1 Kaplan–Meier Curve   84
         7.1.2 Log-Rank Test   85
     7.2 Parametric Regression for Censored Data   87
         7.2.1 Linear Regression with Censored Data*   87
         7.2.2 Cox Proportional Hazard Regression   89
         7.2.3 Reanalysis of the Western Collaborative Group Study Data   91

8 Analysis of Censored Data: Survival Trees   93
     8.1 Splitting Criteria   93
         8.1.1 Gordon and Olshen's Rule*   93
         8.1.2 Maximizing the Difference   96
         8.1.3 Use of Likelihood Functions*   96
         8.1.4 A Straightforward Extension   99
     8.2 Pruning a Survival Tree   99
     8.3 Implementation   100
     8.4 Survival Trees for the Western Collaborative Group Study Data   101

9 Regression Trees and Adaptive Splines for a Continuous Response • 105
9.1 Tree Representation of Spline Model and Analysis of Birth Weight 106
9.2 Regression Trees 108
9.3 The Profile of MARS Models 112
9.4 Modified MARS Forward Procedure 115
9.5 MARS Backward-Deletion Step 118
9.6 The Best Knot* 120
9.7 Restrictions on the Knot* 123
    9.7.1 Minimum Span 123
    9.7.2 Maximal Correlation 124
    9.7.3 Patches to the MARS Forward Algorithm 127
9.8 Smoothing Adaptive Splines* 127
    9.8.1 Smoothing the Linearly Truncated Basis Functions . 128
    9.8.2 Cubic Basis Functions 128
9.9 Numerical Examples 129

10 Analysis of Longitudinal Data • 137
10.1 Infant Growth Curves 137
10.2 The Notation and a General Model 139
10.3 Mixed-Effects Models 140
10.4 Semiparametric Models 143
10.5 Adaptive Spline Models 144
    10.5.1 Known Covariance Structure 145
    10.5.2 Unknown Covariance Structure 146
    10.5.3 A Simulated Example 149
    10.5.4 Reanalyses of Two Published Data Sets 152
    10.5.5 Analysis of Infant Growth Curves 161
    10.5.6 Remarks 166
10.6 Regression Trees for Longitudinal Data 167
    10.6.1 Example: HIV in San Francisco 169

11 Analysis of Multiple Discrete Responses • 173
11.1 Parametric Methods for Binary Responses 175
    11.1.1 Log-Linear Models 176
    11.1.2 Marginal Models 178
    11.1.3 Parameter Estimation* 179
    11.1.4 Frailty Models 181
11.2 Classification Trees for Multiple Binary Responses 183
    11.2.1 Within-Node Homogeneity 183
    11.2.2 Terminal Nodes 184
    11.2.3 Computational Issues* 185
    11.2.4 Parameter Interpretation* 186
11.3 Application: Analysis of BROCS Data 187

	11.3.1	Background	187
	11.3.2	Tree Construction	189
	11.3.3	Description of Numerical Results	192
	11.3.4	Alternative Approaches	192
	11.3.5	Predictive Performance	193
11.4	Polytomous and Longitudinal Responses	195
11.5	Analysis of the BROCS Data via Log-Linear Models	195

12 Appendix   201

    12.1 The Script for Running RTREE Automatically 201
    12.2 The Script for Running RTREE Manually 203
    12.3 The `.inf` File 207

References   211

Index   223

1
Introduction

Many scientific problems reduce to modeling the relationship between two sets of variables. Regression methodology is designed to quantify these relationships. *Recursive Partitioning* is a statistical technique that forms the basis for two classes of nonparametric regression methods: Classification and Regression Trees (CART) and Multivariate Adaptive Regression Splines (MARS). Although relatively new, these methods have a growing number of applications, particularly in the health sciences, as a result of increasing complexity of study designs and data structures.

Due to their mathematical simplicity, linear regression for continuous data, logistic regression for binary data, proportional hazard regression for censored survival data, and mixed-effect regression for longitudinal data are among the most commonly used statistical methods. These parametric regression methods, however, may not lead to faithful data descriptions when the underlying assumptions are not satisfied. Sometimes, model interpretation can be problematic in the presence of higher-order interactions among potent predictors.

Nonparametric regression has evolved to relax or remove the restrictive assumptions. In many cases, recursive partitioning is used to explore data structures and to derive parsimonious models. The theme of this book is to describe nonparametric regression methods built on recursive partitioning. While explaining the methodology in its entirety, we emphasize the applications of these methods in the health sciences. Moreover, it should become apparent from these applications that the resulting models have very natural and useful interpretations, and the computation will be less and less an issue. Specifically, we will see that the tree representations can be stated as a string of hierarchal Boolean statements, facilitating conversion of complex output to narrative form.

In Section 1.1 we give a number of examples for which recursive partitioning has been used to investigate a broad spectrum of scientific problems. In Section 1.2 we formulate these scientific problems into a general regression framework and introduce the necessary notation. To conclude this chapter, we outline the contents of the subsequent chapters in Section 1.3.

1.1 Examples Using CART

Recursive partitioning has been applied to understand many clinical problems. The examples selected below are not necessarily fully representative, but they give us some idea about the breadth of applications.

Example 1.1 Goldman et al. (1982, 1996) provided a classic example of using CART. Their purpose was to build an expert computer system that could assist physicians in emergency rooms to classify patients with chest pain into relatively homogeneous groups within a few hours of admission using the clinical factors available. This classification can help physicians to plan for appropriate levels of medical care for patients based on their classified group membership. The authors included 10,682 patients with acute chest pain in the derivation data set and 4,676 in the validation data set. The derivation data were used to set up a basic model frame, while the validation data were utilized to justify the model and to conduct hypothesis testing.

Example 1.2 Levy et al. (1985) carried out one of the early applications of CART. To predict the outcome from coma caused by cerebral hypoxia-ischemia, they studied 210 patients with cerebral hypoxia-ischemia and considered 13 factors including age, sex, verbal and motor responses, and eye opening movement. Several guidelines were derived to predict within the first few days which patients would do well and which would do poorly.

Example 1.3 Mammalian sperm move in distinctive patterns, called hyperactivated motility, during capacitation. Figure 1.1(a) is a circular pattern of hyperactivated rabbit spermatozoa, and Figure 1.1(b) displays a nonhyperactivated track. In general, hyperactivated motility is characterized by a change from progressive movement to highly vigorous, nonprogressive random motion. This motility is useful for the investigation of sperm function and the assessment of fertility. For this reason, we must establish a quantitative criterion that recognizes hyperactivated sperm in a mixed population of hyperactivated and nonhyperactivated sperm. After collecting 322 hyperactivated and 899 nonhyperactivated sperm, Young and Bod (1994) derived a classification rule based on the wobble parameter of motility and the curvilinear velocity, using CART. Their rule was shown

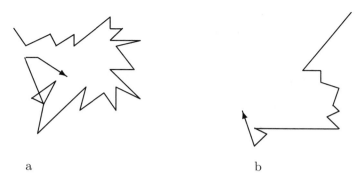

FIGURE 1.1. Motility patterns for mammalian sperm. (a) Hyperactivated and (b) nonhyperactivated.

to have a lower misclassification rate than the commonly used ones that were established by linear discriminant analysis.

Example 1.4 Important medical decisions are commonly made while substantial uncertainty remains. Acute unexplained fever in infants is one of such frequently encountered problems. To make a correct diagnosis, it is critical to utilize information efficiently, including medical history, physical examination, and laboratory tests. Using a sample of 1,218 childhood extremity injuries seen in 1987 and 1988 by residents in family medicine and pediatrics in the Rochester General Hospital Emergency Department, McConnochie, Roghmann, and Pasternack (1993) demonstrated the value of the complementary use of logistic regression and CART in developing clinical guidelines.

Example 1.5 Birth weight and gestational age are strong predictors for neonatal mortality and morbidity; see, e.g., Bracken (1984). In less developed countries, however, birth weight may not be measured for the first time until several days after birth, by which time substantial weight loss could have occurred. There are also practical problems in those countries in obtaining gestational age because many illiterate pregnant women cannot record the dates of their last menstrual period or calculate the duration of gestational age. For these considerations, Raymond et al. (1994) selected 843 singleton infants born at a referral hospital in Addis Ababa, Ethiopia, in 1987 and 1988 and applied CART to build a practical screening tool based on neonatal body measurements that are presumably more stable than birth weight. Their study suggests that head and chest circumferences may predict adequately the risk of low birth weight (less than 2,500 grams) and preterm (less than 37 weeks of gestational age) delivery.

Example 1.6 Head injuries cause about a half million patient hospitalizations in the United States each year. As a result of the injury, victims often suffer from persistent disabilities. It is of profound clinical importance to make early prediction of long-term outcome so that the patient, the family, and the physicians have sufficient time to arrange a suitable rehabilitation plan. Moreover, this outcome prediction can also provide useful information for assessing the treatment effect. Using CART, Choi et al. (1991) and Temkin et al. (1995) have developed prediction rules for long-term outcome in patients with head injuries on the basis of 514 patients. Those rules are simple and accurate enough for clinical practice.

1.2 The Statistical Problem

Examples 1.1–1.6 can be summarized into the same statistical problem as follows. They all have an outcome variable, Y, and a set of p predictors, $x_1, \ldots, x_p$. The number of predictors, p, varies from example to example. The x's will be regarded as fixed variables, and Y is a random variable. In example 1.3, Y is a dichotomous variable representing either hyperactivated or nonhyperactivated sperm. The x's include the wobble parameter of motility and the curvilinear velocity. Obviously, not all predictors appear in the prediction rule. Likewise, the x's and Y can be easily identified for the other examples. The statistical problem is to establish a relationship between Y and the x's so that it is possible to predict Y based on the values of the x's. Mathematically, we want to estimate the conditional probability of the random variable Y,

$$I\!\!P\{Y = y \,|\, x_1, \ldots, x_p\}, \tag{1.1}$$

or a functional of this probability such as the conditional expectation

$$I\!\!E\{Y \,|\, x_1, \ldots, x_p\}. \tag{1.2}$$

Since Examples 1.1–1.6 involve dichotomous Y (0 or 1), the conditional expectation in (1.2) coincides with the conditional probability in (1.1) with $y = 1$. In such circumstances, logistic regression is commonly used, assuming that the conditional probability (1.1) is of a specific form,

$$\frac{\exp(\beta_0 + \sum_{i=1}^{p} \beta_i x_i)}{1 + \exp(\beta_0 + \sum_{i=1}^{p} \beta_i x_i)}, \tag{1.3}$$

where the β's are parameters to be estimated.

In the ordinary linear regression, the conditional probability in (1.1) is assumed to be a normal density function,

$$\frac{1}{\sqrt{2\pi}} \exp\left[-\frac{(y-\mu)^2}{2\sigma^2}\right], \tag{1.4}$$

TABLE 1.1. Correspondence Between the Uses of Classic Approaches and Recursive Partitioning Technique in This Book

Type of response	Parametric methods	Recursive partitioning technique
Continuous	Ordinary linear regression	Regression trees and adaptive splines in Chapter 9
Binary	Logistic regression in Chapter 3	Classification trees in Chapter 4
Censored	Proportion hazard regression in Chapter 7	Survival trees in Chapter 8
Longitudinal	Mixed-effects models in Chapter 10	Regression trees and adaptive splines in Chapter 10
Multiple discrete	Exponential, marginal, and frailty models	Classification trees, all in Chapter 11

where the mean, μ, equals the conditional expectation in (1.2) and is of a hypothesized expression

$$\mu = \beta_0 + \sum_{i=1}^{p} \beta_i x_i. \qquad (1.5)$$

The σ^2 in (1.4) is an unknown variance parameter. We use $N(\mu, \sigma^2)$ to denote the normal distribution corresponding to the density in (1.4).

In contrast to these models, recursive partitioning is a nonparametric technique that does not require a specified model structure like (1.3) or (1.5). In the subsequent chapters, the outcome Y may represent a censored measurement or a correlated set of responses. We will cite more examples accordingly.

1.3 Outline of the Methodology

In this book, we will describe both classic (mostly parametric) and modern statistical techniques as complementary tools for the analysis of data in the health sciences. The five types of response variables listed in Table 1.1 cover the majority of the data that arise from health-related studies. Table 1.1 conforms with the content of this book. Thus, it is not a complete list of methods that are available in the literature.

Chapter 2 is a practical guide to tree construction, focusing on the statistical ideas and scientific judgment. Technical details are deferred to Chapter 4, where methodological issues involved in classification trees are discussed in depth. We refer to Breiman et al. (1984) for further elaboration. Section 4.2.3 on *Nested Optimal Subtrees* is relatively technical and may be difficult for some readers, but the rest of Chapter 4 is relatively straightforward. Technical differences between classification trees and regression trees are very minimal. After elucidating classification trees in Chapter 4, we introduce regression trees briefly, but sufficiently, in Section 9.2, focusing on the differences. To further demonstrate the use of classification trees, we report a stratified tree-based risk factor analysis of spontaneous abortion in Chapter 5.

Chapters 6 to 8 cover the analysis of censored data. The first part is a shortcut to the output of survival trees. We present classical methods of survival analysis prior to the exposition of survival trees in the last compartment of this coverage.

Chapter 11 on classification trees for multiple binary responses is nearly parallel to survival trees from a methodological point of view. Thus, they can be read separately depending on the different needs of readers.

We start a relatively distinct topic in Chapter 9 that is fundamental to the understanding of adaptive regression splines and should be read before Chapter 10, where the use of adaptive splines is further expanded.

Before discussing the trees and splines approaches, we will describe their parametric counterparts and explain how to use these more standard models. We view it as important to understand and appreciate the parametric methods even though the main topic of this book is recursive partitioning.

2
A Practical Guide to Tree Construction

We introduce the basic ideas associated with recursive partitioning in the context of a specific scientific question: Which pregnant women are most at risk of preterm deliveries? Particular emphasis is placed on the interaction between scientific judgment by investigators and the production of informative intermediate-stage computer output that facilitates the generation of the most sensible recursive partitioning trees.

The illustrative database is the Yale Pregnancy Outcome Study, a project funded by the National Institutes of Health, and it has been under the leadership of Dr. Michael B. Bracken at Yale University. The study subjects were women who made a first prenatal visit to a private obstetrics or midwife practice, health maintenance organization, or hospital clinic in the greater New Haven, Connecticut, area between May 12, 1980, and March 12, 1982, and who anticipated delivery at the Yale–New Haven Hospital. For illustration, we take a subset of 3,861 women from this database by selecting those women whose pregnancies ended in a singleton live birth and who met the eligibility criteria for inclusion as specified in detail by Bracken et al. (1986) and Zhang and Bracken (1995).

Preterm delivery will be the outcome variable of interest. Based on the extant literature, Zhang and Bracken (1995) considered 15 variables a priori as candidates to be useful in representing routes to preterm delivery. The variables are listed in Table 2.1.

TABLE 2.1. A List of Candidate Predictor Variables

Variable name	Label	Type	Range/levels
Maternal age	x_1	Continuous	13–46
Marital status	x_2	Nominal	Currently married, divorced, separated, widowed, never married
Race	x_3	Nominal	White, Black, Hispanic, Asian, others
Marijuana use	x_4	Nominal	Yes, no
Times of using marijuana	x_5	Ordinal	>= 5, 3–4, 2, 1 (daily) 4–6, 1–3 (weekly) 2–3, 1, < 1 (monthly)
Years of education	x_6	Continuous	4–27
Employment	x_7	Nominal	Yes, no
Smoker	x_8	Nominal	Yes, no
Cigarettes smoked	x_9	Continuous	0–66
Passive smoking	x_{10}	Nominal	Yes, no
Gravidity	x_{11}	Ordinal	1–10
Hormones/DES used by mother	x_{12}	Nominal	None, hormones, DES, both, uncertain
Alcohol (oz/day)	x_{13}	Ordinal	0–3
Caffeine (mg)	x_{14}	Continuous	12.6–1273
Parity	x_{15}	Ordinal	0–7

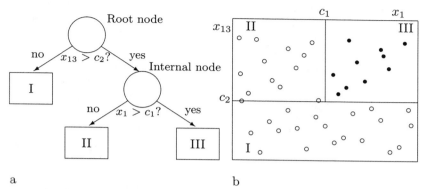

a   b

FIGURE 2.1. An illustrative tree structure. x_1 is age and x_{13} is the amount of alcohol drinking. Circles and dots are different outcomes.

2.1 The Elements of Tree Construction

To pin down the basic ideas, consider the simple tree diagram in Figure 2.1. The tree has three layers of nodes. The first layer is the unique root node, namely, the circle on the top. One internal (the circle) node is in the second layer, and three terminal (the boxes) nodes are respectively in the second and third layers. Here, the root node can also be regarded as an internal node. Both the root and the internal nodes are partitioned into two nodes in the next layer that are called left and right daughter nodes. By definition, however, the terminal nodes do not have offspring nodes.

To understand the construction of Figure 2.1, we need to answer three basic questions:

- What are the contents of the nodes?
- Why and how is a parent node split into two daughter nodes?
- When do we declare a terminal node?

The root node contains a sample of subjects from which the tree is grown. Those subjects constitute the so-called learning sample, and the learning sample can be the entire study sample or a subset of it. For our example, the root node contains all 3,861 pregnant women who were the study subjects of the Yale Pregnancy Outcome Study. All nodes in the same layer constitute a partition of the root node. The partition becomes finer and finer as the layer gets deeper and deeper. Therefore, every node in a tree is merely a subset of the learning sample.

Figure 2.1(b) illustrates a hypothetical situation. Let a dot denote a preterm delivery and a circle stand for a term delivery. The two coordinates represent two covariates, x_1 (age) and x_{13} (the amount of alcohol drinking), as defined in Table 2.1. We can draw two line segments to separate the dots from the circles and obtain three disjoint regions: (I) $x_{13} \leq c_2$; (II) $x_{13} > c_2$ and $x_1 \leq c_1$; and (III) $x_{13} > c_2$ and $x_1 > c_1$. Thus, partition I is not divided by x_1, and partitions I and II are identical in response but described differently.

In the same figure, panel (a) is a tree representation of this separation. First, we put both the dots and the circles into the root node. The two arrows below the root node direct a dot or circle to terminal node I or the internal node in the second layer, depending on whether or not $x_{13} \leq c_2$. Those with $x_{13} > c_2$ are further directed to terminal nodes II and III based on whether or not $x_1 \leq c_1$. Hence, the nodes in panel (a) correspond to the regions in panel (b). When we draw a line to separate a region, it amounts to partitioning a node in the tree. The precise maps between regions I to III and terminal nodes I to III, respectively, can be found in Figure 2.1.

The essence of recursive partitioning is that the terminal nodes are homogeneous in the sense that they contain either dots or circles. On the other hand, the two internal nodes are heterogeneous because they contain both dots and circles. Because dots and circles represent preterm and term deliveries, respectively, Figure 2.1 would suggest that all pregnant women older than a certain age and drinking more than a certain amount of alcohol daily deliver preterm infants. Consequently, this would demonstrate a hypothetically ideal association of preterm delivery to the age and alcohol consumption of the pregnant women.

Complete homogeneity of terminal nodes is an ideal that is rarely realized. Thus, the numerical objective of partitioning is to make the contents of the terminal nodes as homogeneous as possible. A quantitative measure of the extent of node homogeneity is the notion of node impurity. The simplest operationalization of the idea is:

$$\frac{\text{Number of women having a preterm delivery in a node}}{\text{Total number of women in the node}}.$$

The closer this ratio is to 0 or 1, the more homogeneous is the node.

2.2 Splitting a Node

We focus on the root node and observe that the same process applies to the partition of any node. All allowable splits, with appropriate discretization of continuous variables, are considered for the predictor variables in Table 2.1. To understand the process, let us focus initially on the variable x_1 (age). It has 32 distinct age values in the range of 13 to 46. Hence, it may result in $32 - 1 = 31$ allowable splits. For example, one split can be whether or not age is more than 35 years (i.e., $x_1 > 35$). In general, for an ordinal (e.g., times of using marijuana) or a continuous (e.g., caffeine intake) predictor, x_j, the number of allowable splits is one fewer than the

2.2 Splitting a Node

TABLE 2.2. Allowable Splits Using Race

Left daughter node	Right daughter node
White	Black, Hispanic, Asian, others
Black	White, Hispanic, Asian, others
Hispanic	White, Black, Asian, others
Asian	White, Black, Hispanic, others
White, Black	Hispanic, Asian, others
White, Hispanic	Black, Asian, others
White, Asian	Black, Hispanic, others
Black, Hispanic	White, Asian, others
Black, Asian	White, Hispanic, others
Hispanic, Asian	White, Black, others
Black, Hispanic, Asian	White, others
White, Hispanic, Asian	Black, others
White, Black, Asian	Hispanic, others
White, Black, Hispanic	Asian, others
White, Black, Hispanic, Asian	Others

number of its distinctly observed values. For instance, there are 153 different levels of daily caffeine intake ranging from 0 to 1273 mg in the 3,861 study subjects. Thus, we can split the root node in 152 different ways based on the amount of caffeine intake.

What happens to nominal predictors is slightly more complicated. In Table 2.1, x_3 denotes 5 ethnic groups that do not have a particular order. Table 2.2 lays out $2^{5-1} - 1 = 15$ allowable splits from this ethnicity variable. Generally, any nominal variable that has k levels contributes $2^{k-1} - 1$ allowable splits.

Adding together the numbers of allowable splits from the 15 predictors in Table 2.1, we have 347 possible ways to divide the root node into two subnodes. Depending on the number of the predictors and the nature of the predictors, the total number of the allowable splits for the root node varies, though it is usually not small. The basic question to be addressed now is, How do we select one or several preferred splits from the pool of allowable splits?

Before selecting the best split, we must define the goodness of a split. What we want is a split that results in two pure (or homogeneous) daughter nodes. However, in reality the daughter nodes are usually partially homogeneous. Therefore, the goodness of a split must weigh the homogeneities (or the impurities) in the two daughter nodes. If we take age as a tentative splitting covariate and consider its cutoff at c, as a result of the question "Is $x_1 > c$?" we have the following table:

2. A Practical Guide to Tree Construction

		Term	Preterm	
Left Node (τ_L)	$x_1 \leq c$	n_{11}	n_{12}	$n_{1.}$
Right Node (τ_R)	$x_1 > c$	n_{21}	n_{22}	$n_{2.}$
		$n_{.1}$	$n_{.2}$	

Now let $Y = 1$ if a woman has a preterm delivery and $Y = 0$ otherwise. We estimate $I\!P\{Y = 1|\tau_L\}$ and $I\!P\{Y = 1|\tau_R\}$ by $n_{12}/n_{1.}$ and $n_{22}/n_{2.}$, respectively. Introduce the notion of entropy impurity in the left daughter node as

$$i(\tau_L) = -\frac{n_{11}}{n_{1.}} \log\left(\frac{n_{11}}{n_{1.}}\right) - \frac{n_{12}}{n_{1.}} \log\left(\frac{n_{12}}{n_{1.}}\right). \qquad (2.1)$$

Likewise, define the impurity in the right daughter node as

$$i(\tau_R) = -\frac{n_{21}}{n_{2.}} \log\left(\frac{n_{21}}{n_{2.}}\right) - \frac{n_{22}}{n_{2.}} \log\left(\frac{n_{22}}{n_{2.}}\right). \qquad (2.2)$$

Then, the goodness of a split, s, is measured by

$$\Delta I(s,\tau) = i(\tau) - I\!P\{\tau_L\}i(\tau_L) - I\!P\{\tau_R\}i(\tau_R), \qquad (2.3)$$

where τ is the parent of τ_L and τ_R, and $I\!P\{\tau_L\}$ and $I\!P\{\tau_R\}$ are respectively the probabilities that a subject falls into nodes τ_L and τ_R. At present, $I\!P\{\tau_L\}$ can be replaced with $n_{1.}/(n_{1.}+n_{2.})$ and $I\!P\{\tau_R\}$ with $n_{2.}/(n_{1.}+n_{2.})$.

The criterion (2.3) measures the degree of reduction in the impurity by going from the parent node to the daughter nodes.

To appreciate these concepts in more detail, let us go through a concrete example. If we take $c = 35$ as the age threshold, we have a 2×2 table

	Term	Preterm	
Left Node (τ_L)	3521	198	3719
Right Node (τ_R)	135	7	142
	3656	205	3861

Then, $i(\tau_L)$ in (2.1) equals

$$-(3521/3719)\log(3521/3719) - (198/3719)\log(198/3719) = 0.2079.$$

Similarly, $i(\tau_R)$ in (2.2) is 0.1964, and $i(\tau) = 0.20753$. Substituting these impurities into (2.3), we have $\Delta I(s,\tau) = 0.00001$.

We know that there are 31 allowable age splits. Table 2.3 reports $\Delta I(s,\tau)$ for all allowable age splits. From Table 2.3, we see that the greatest reduction in the impurity comes from the age split at 24. This table is an important piece of output for an investigator to examine. In particular, it might be judged to be more interesting to force an age split at age 19, stratifying the study sample into teenagers and adults. This is tantamount to selecting the second-best split by our numerical criterion while using scientific judgment in a decisive manner to overrule the automated procedure. We view

TABLE 2.3. The Goodness of Allowable Age Splits

Split value	Impurity Left node	Right node	1000*Goodness of the split (1000Δ)
13	0.00000	0.20757	0.01
14	0.00000	0.20793	0.14
15	0.31969	0.20615	0.17
16	0.27331	0.20583	0.13
17	0.27366	0.20455	0.23
18	0.31822	0.19839	1.13
19	0.30738	0.19508	1.40
20	0.28448	0.19450	1.15
21	0.27440	0.19255	1.15
22	0.26616	0.18965	1.22
23	0.25501	0.18871	1.05
(24)	0.25747	0.18195	(1.50)
25	0.24160	0.18479	0.92
26	0.23360	0.18431	0.72
27	0.22750	0.18344	0.58
28	0.22109	0.18509	0.37
29	0.21225	0.19679	0.06
30	0.20841	0.20470	0.00
31	0.20339	0.22556	0.09
32	0.20254	0.23871	0.18
33	0.20467	0.23524	0.09
34	0.20823	0.19491	0.01
35	0.20795	0.19644	0.01
36	0.20744	0.21112	0.00
37	0.20878	0.09804	0.18
38	0.20857	0.00000	0.37
39	0.20805	0.00000	0.18
40	0.20781	0.00000	0.10
41	0.20769	0.00000	0.06
42	0.20761	0.00000	0.03
43	0.20757	0.00000	0.01

TABLE 2.4. The Largest Goodness of Split from All Predictors

Variable	x_1	x_2	x_3	x_4	x_5	x_6	x_7	x_8
$1000\Delta I$	1.5	2.8	4.0	0.6	0.6	3.2	0.7	0.6
Variable	x_9	x_{10}	x_{11}	x_{12}	x_{13}	x_{14}	x_{15}	
$1000\Delta I$	0.7	0.2	1.8	1.1	0.5	0.8	1.2	

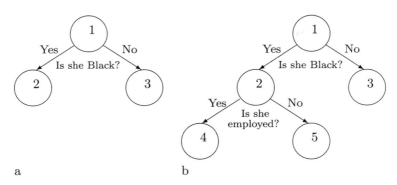

FIGURE 2.2. Node splitting, recursive partitioning process. Node 1 is split into nodes 2 and 3 and then node 2 into nodes 4 and 5.

this kind of interactive process as fundamentally important in producing the most interpretable trees.

This best or preferred age split is used to compete with the best (or respectively preferred) splits from the other 14 predictors. Table 2.4 presents the greatest numerical goodness of split for all predictors. We see that the best of the best comes from the race variable with $1000\Delta I = 4.0$, i.e., $\Delta I = 0.004$. This best split divides the root node according to whether a pregnant woman is Black or not. This partition is illustrated in Figure 2.2(a), where the root node (number 1) is split into nodes 2 (Black) and 3 (non-Black).

After splitting the root node, we continue to divide its two daughter nodes. The partitioning principle is the same. For example, to further divide node 2 in Figure 2.2(b) into nodes 4 and 5, we repeat the previous partitioning process with a minor adjustment. That is, the partition uses only 710 Black women, and the remaining 3,151 non-Black women are put aside. The pool of allowable splits is nearly intact except that race does not contribute any more splits, as everyone is now Black. So, the total number of allowable splits decreases from 347 to at least 332. It is useful to notice the decreasing trend of the number of allowable splits, but it is not important for us to know the precise counts. After the split of node 2, we have three nodes (numbers 3, 4, and 5) ready to be split. In the same way, we can divide node 3 in Figure 2.2(b) as we did for node 2. But remember that this time we consider only the 3,151 non-Black women. Furthermore, there are potentially $2^{4-1} - 1 = 7$ race splits because the category of non-Black women comprises Whites, Hispanics, Asians, and other ethnic groups. Hence, there can be as many as 339 allowable splits for node 3. One important message is that an offspring node may use the same splitting variable as its ancestors. After we finish node 3, we go on to nodes 4 and 5, and so on. This is the so-called *recursive partitioning* process. Because we partition one node into two nodes only, the resulting tree is called a binary tree.

2.3 Terminal Nodes

The recursive partitioning process may proceed until the tree is saturated in the sense that the offspring nodes subject to further division cannot be split. This happens, for instance, when there is only one subject in a node. Note that the total number of allowable splits for a node drops as we move from one layer to the next. As a result, the number of allowable splits eventually reduces to zero, and the tree cannot be split any further. Any node that we cannot or will not split is a terminal node. The saturated tree is usually too large to be useful, because the terminal nodes are so small that we cannot make sensible statistical inference; and this level of detail is rarely scientifically interpretable. It is typically unnecessary to wait until the tree is saturated. Instead, a minimum size of a node is set a priori. We stop splitting when a node is smaller than the minimum. The choice of the minimum size depends on the sample size (e.g., one percent) or can be simply taken as 5 subjects (the results are generally not so meaningful with fewer than 5 subjects).

During the early development of recursive partitioning, stopping rules were proposed to quit the partitioning process before the tree becomes too large. For example, the Automatic Interaction Detection (AID) program proposed by Morgan and Sonquist (1963) declares a terminal node based on the relative merit of its best split to the quality of the root node.

Breiman et al. (1984, p. 37) argued that depending on the stopping threshold, the partitioning tends to end too soon or too late. Accordingly, they made a fundamental shift by introducing a second step, called pruning. Instead of attempting to stop the partitioning, they propose to let the partitioning continue until it is saturated or nearly so. Beginning with this generally large tree, we prune it from the bottom up. The point is to find a subtree of the saturated tree that is most "predictive" of the outcome and least vulnerable to the noise in the data. This is a sophisticated process, and it will be delineated in Chapter 4.

The partitioning and pruning steps can be viewed as variants of forward and backward stepwise procedures in linear regression. The partition of a node in a tree amounts to the addition of a new term to a linear model. Likewise, pruning some nodes at the bottom of a tree corresponds to deleting a few terms from a linear model.

2.4 Download and Use of Software

A standalone commercial program called CART can be purchased from Salford Systems for the analysis of single-response data. Other more standard statistical software such as SPLUS and SPSS also provide tree construction procedures with user-friendly graphical interface. Various related computer programs are freely available for performing most of the data analyses in this book. Most of them can be downloaded from Heping Zhang's web site: http://peace.med.yale.edu/pub. Those who do not have access to the Internet can send their requests to him.

After the program called RTREE is downloaded, it is immediately executable. RTREE can be run in either of two modes: automatic or manual. We recommend running the automatic mode first to product a tree sketch, which then can be used as the reference to run the manual mode. Chapter 12 (the appendix) provides detailed information on the use of this program.

Figure 2.3 is a tree produced automatically by the computer following the ideas described above and the details in Chapter 4. Let us examine the 2,980 non-Black women who had no more than 4 pregnancies. The split for this group of women is based on their mothers' use of hormones and/or DES. If their mothers used hormones and/or DES, or the answers were not reported, they are assigned to the left daughter node. The right daughter node consists of those women whose mothers did not use hormones or DES, or who reported uncertainty about their mothers' use. Thus, women with the "uncertain" answer and the missing answer are assigned to different sides of the parent node although these two types of answers are practically the same. To resolve this conflict, we can force the women with missing answers to the same node as those who answered "uncertain." To do so, we need to manually change the split. Numerically, the goodness of split, Δ, changes from 0.00176 to 0.00148. This leads to the tree in Figure 2.4.

The tree in Figure 2.4 is also smaller than the one in Figure 2.3. This is because the further pruned nodes are less stable, and the significance of the corresponding splits lacks justification. The relative risk and its confidence interval reported for each split are calculated using a cross-validation procedure, as will be elaborated in Section 4.6.

The principal features of Figure 2.4 answer the original question about which pregnant women are most at risk of preterm delivery: (a) Non-Black women who have 4 or fewer prior pregnancies and whose mothers used DES and/or other hormones are at highest risk. In particular, 19.4% of these women have preterm deliveries as opposed to 3.8% whose mothers did not use DES; and (b) Among Black women who are also unemployed, 11.5% had preterm deliveries, as opposed to 5.5% among employed Black women.

The changes that we made to Figure 2.3 are limited for illustrative purposes. One may probe the tree further and find some other trees worth examining. For example, employment status may just serve as a proxy for

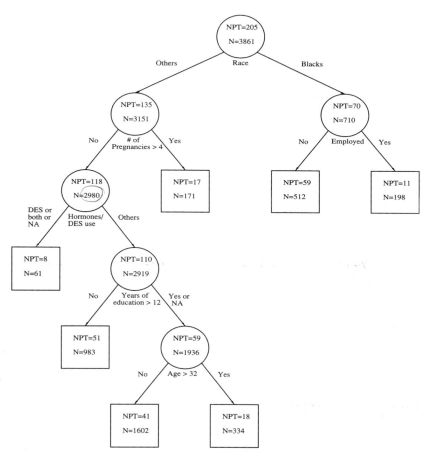

FIGURE 2.3. The computer-selected tree structure. N: sample size; NPT: number of preterm cases.

18   2. A Practical Guide to Tree Construction

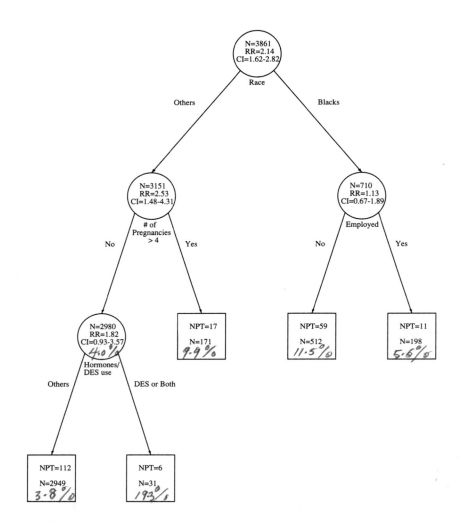

FIGURE 2.4. The final tree structure. N: sample size; RR: relative risk estimated by cross-validation; CI: 95% confidence interval; NPT: number of preterm cases.

more biological circumstances. We can replace it with related biological measures if they are actually available. Zhang (1998b) presents another interesting example of altering the splits of various nodes—a process called swapping by Chipman, George, and McCulloch (1998)—in order to achieve a higher precision of tumor classification.

3
Logistic Regression

We have seen from Examples 1.1–1.6 that the status of many health conditions is represented by a binary response. Because of its practical importance, analyzing a binary response has been the subject of countless works; see, e.g., the books of Cox (1989), Agresti (1990), and the references therein. For comparison purposes, we give a brief introduction to logistic regression.

3.1 Logistic Regression Models

Logistic regression is a standard approach to the analysis of binary data. For every study subject i we assume that the response Y_i has the Bernoulli distribution

$$I\!P\{Y_i = y_i\} = \theta_i^{y_i}(1-\theta_i)^{1-y_i}, \quad y_i = 0, 1, \; i = 1, \ldots, n, \qquad (3.1)$$

where the parameters

$$\boldsymbol{\theta} = (\theta_1, \ldots, \theta_n)'$$

must be estimated from the data. Here, a prime denotes the transpose of a vector or matrix.

To model these data, we generally attempt to reduce the n parameters in $\boldsymbol{\theta}$ to fewer degrees of freedom. The unique feature of logistic regression is to accomplish this by introducing the logit link function:

$$\theta_i = \frac{\exp(\beta_0 + \sum_{j=1}^{p} \beta_j x_{ij})}{1 + \exp(\beta_0 + \sum_{j=1}^{p} \beta_j x_{ij})}, \qquad (3.2)$$

where
$$\boldsymbol{\beta} = (\beta_0, \beta_1, \ldots, \beta_p)'$$
is the new $(p+1)$-vector of parameters to be estimated and $(x_{i1}, \ldots, x_{ip})$ are the values of the p covariates included in the model for the ith subject $(i = 1, \ldots, n)$.

To estimate $\boldsymbol{\beta}$, we make use of the likelihood function

$$\begin{aligned} L(\boldsymbol{\beta}; \mathbf{y}) &= \prod_{i=1}^{n} \left[\frac{\exp(\beta_0 + \sum_{j=1}^{p} \beta_j x_{ij})}{1 + \exp(\beta_0 + \sum_{j=1}^{p} \beta_j x_{ij})} \right]^{y_i} \left[\frac{1}{1 + \exp(\beta_0 + \sum_{j=1}^{p} \beta_j x_{ij})} \right]^{1-y_i} \\ &= \frac{\prod_{y_i=1} \exp(\beta_0 + \sum_{j=1}^{p} \beta_j x_{ij})}{\prod_{i=1}^{n} [1 + \exp(\beta_0 + \sum_{j=1}^{p} \beta_j x_{ij})]}. \end{aligned}$$

By maximizing $L(\boldsymbol{\beta}; \mathbf{y})$, we obtain the maximum likelihood estimate $\hat{\boldsymbol{\beta}}$ of $\boldsymbol{\beta}$. Although the solution for $\hat{\boldsymbol{\beta}}$ is unique, it does not have a closed form. The Newton–Raphson method, an iterative algorithm, computes $\hat{\boldsymbol{\beta}}$ numerically; see, e.g., Agresti (1990, Section 4.7).

The interpretation of the parameter $\boldsymbol{\beta}$ is the most attractive feature of the logit link function. Based on (3.2), the odds that the ith subject has an abnormal condition is

$$\frac{\theta_i}{1 - \theta_i} = \exp\left(\beta_0 + \sum_{j=1}^{p} \beta_j x_{ij}\right).$$

Consider two individuals i and k for whom $x_{i1} = 1$, $x_{k1} = 0$, and $x_{ij} = x_{kj}$ for $j = 2, \ldots, p$. Then, the odds ratio for subjects i and k to be abnormal is

$$\frac{\theta_i/(1-\theta_i)}{\theta_k/(1-\theta_k)} = \exp(\beta_1).$$

Taking the logarithm of both sides, we see that β_1 is the log odds ratio of the response resulting from two such subjects when their first covariate differs by one unit and the other covariates are the same. In the health sciences, $\exp(\beta_1)$ is referred to as the adjusted odds ratio attributed to x_1 while controlling for $x_2, \ldots, x_p$. The remaining β's have similar interpretations. This useful interpretation may become invalid, however, in the presence of interactive effects among covariates.

3.2 A Logistic Regression Analysis

In this section we analyze the Yale Pregnancy Outcome data using logistic regression. Most statistical packages include procedures for logistic regression. We used SAS to perform the analysis. First, we start with a model that

3.2 A Logistic Regression Analysis

includes all predictors in Table 2.1 as main effects and use the backward stepwise procedure to select variables that have significant (at the level of 0.05) main effects. Recall that preterm delivery is our response variable. For the selected variables, we then consider their second-order interactions.

In Table 2.1, three predictors, x_2 (marital status), x_3 (race), and x_{12} (hormones/DES use), are nominal and have five levels. To include them in logistic regression models, we need to create four (dichotomous) dummy variables for each of them. For instance, Table 2.1 indicates that the five levels for x_2 are currently married, divorced, separated, widowed, and never married. Let

$$z_1 = \begin{cases} 1 & \text{if a subject was currently married,} \\ 0 & \text{otherwise,} \end{cases}$$

$$z_2 = \begin{cases} 1 & \text{if a subject was divorced,} \\ 0 & \text{otherwise,} \end{cases}$$

$$z_3 = \begin{cases} 1 & \text{if a subject was separated,} \\ 0 & \text{otherwise,} \end{cases}$$

$$z_4 = \begin{cases} 1 & \text{if a subject was widowed,} \\ 0 & \text{otherwise.} \end{cases}$$

Likewise, let

$$z_5 = \begin{cases} 1 & \text{for a Caucasian,} \\ 0 & \text{otherwise,} \end{cases}$$

$$z_6 = \begin{cases} 1 & \text{for an African-American,} \\ 0 & \text{otherwise,} \end{cases}$$

$$z_7 = \begin{cases} 1 & \text{for a Hispanic,} \\ 0 & \text{otherwise,} \end{cases}$$

$$z_8 = \begin{cases} 1 & \text{for an Asian,} \\ 0 & \text{otherwise,} \end{cases}$$

and

$$z_9 = \begin{cases} 1 & \text{if a subject's mother did not use hormones or DES,} \\ 0 & \text{otherwise,} \end{cases}$$

$$z_{10} = \begin{cases} 1 & \text{if a subject's mother used hormones only,} \\ 0 & \text{otherwise,} \end{cases}$$

$$z_{11} = \begin{cases} 1 & \text{if a subject's mother used DES only,} \\ 0 & \text{otherwise,} \end{cases}$$

$$z_{12} = \begin{cases} 1 & \text{if a subject's mother used both hormones and DES,} \\ 0 & \text{otherwise.} \end{cases}$$

Note here that the subject refers to a pregnant woman. Thus, z_9 through z_{12} indicate the history of hormones and DES uses for the mother of a pregnant woman.

3. Logistic Regression

TABLE 3.1. MLE for an Initially Selected Model

Selected variable	Degrees of freedom	Coefficient Estimate	Standard Error	p-value
Intercept	1	−2.172	0.6912	0.0017
x_1(age)	1	0.046	0.0218	0.0356
z_6(Black)	1	0.771	0.2296	0.0008
x_6(educ.)	1	−0.159	0.0501	0.0015
z_{10}(horm.)	1	1.794	0.5744	0.0018

TABLE 3.2. MLE for a Revised Model

Selected variable	Degrees of freedom	Coefficient Estimate	Standard Error	p-value
Intercept	1	−2.334	0.4583	0.0001
x_6(educ.)	1	−0.076	0.0313	0.0151
z_6(Black)	1	0.705	0.1688	0.0001
x_{11}(grav.)	1	0.114	0.0466	0.0142
z_{10}(horm.)	1	1.535	0.4999	0.0021

Due to missing information, 1,797 of the 3,861 observations are not used in the backward deletion step by SAS PROC LOGISTIC. Table 3.1 provides the key information for the model that is selected by the backward stepwise procedure. In this table as well as the next two, the first column refers to the selected predictors, and the second column is the degrees of freedom (DF). The third column contains the estimated coefficients corresponding to selected predictors, followed by the standard errors of the estimated coefficients. The last column gives the p-value for testing whether or not each coefficient is zero. We should note that our model selection used each dummy variable as an individual predictor in the model. As a consequence, the selected model may depend on how the dummy variables are coded. Alternatively, one may want to include or exclude a chunk of dummy variables that are created for the same nominal variable.

The high proportion of the removed observations due to the missing information is an obvious concern. Note that the model selection is based on the observations with complete information in all predictors even though fewer predictors are considered in later steps. We examined the distribution of missing data and removed x_7 (employment) and x_8 (smoking) from further consideration because they were not selected in the first place and they contained most of the missing data. After this strategic adjustment, only 24 observations are removed due to missing data, and the backward deletion process produces another set of variables as displayed in Table 3.2.

We have considered the main effects, and next we examine possible (second-order) interactions between the selected variables. For the two se-

TABLE 3.3. MLE for the Final Model

Selected variable	Degrees of freedom	Coefficient Estimate	Standard Error	p-value
Intercept	1	-2.344	0.4584	0.0001
x_6(educ.)	1	-0.076	0.0313	0.0156
z_6(Black)	1	0.699	0.1688	0.0001
x_{11}(grav.)	1	0.115	0.0466	0.0137
z_{10} (horm.)	1	1.539	0.4999	0.0021

lected dummy variables, we include their original variables, race and hormones/DES uses, into the backward stepwise process to open our eyes a little wider. It turns out that none of the interaction terms are significant at the level of 0.05. Thus, the final model includes the same four variables as those in Table 3.2. However, the estimates in Table 3.2 are based on 3,837 (i.e., 3861 − 24) observations with complete information for 13 predictors. Table 3.3 presents the information for the final model for which only 3 observations are removed due to missing information in the four selected variables. The different numbers of used observations explain the minor numerical discrepancy between Tables 3.2 and 3.3.

From Table 3.3, we see that the odds ratio for a Black woman (z_6) to deliver a premature infant is doubled relative to that for a White woman, because the corresponding odds ratio equals $\exp(0.699) \approx 2.013$. The use of DES by the mother of the pregnant woman (z_{10}) has a significant and enormous effect on the preterm delivery. Years of education (x_6), however, seems to have a small, but significant, protective effect. Finally, the number of previous pregnancies (x_{11}) has a significant, but low-magnitude negative effect on the preterm delivery.

We have witnessed in our analysis that missing data may lead to serious loss of information. As a potential consequence, we may end up with imprecise or even false conclusions. For example, by reviewing Tables 3.1 and 3.3, we realize that x_1 is replaced with x_{11} in Table 3.3 and the estimated coefficients for the remaining three predictors are notably different. The difference could be more dramatic if we had a smaller sample. Therefore, precaution should be taken in the presence of missing data. In Section 4.8, we will see that the tree-based method handles the missing data efficiently by either creating a distinct category for the missing value or using surrogate variables. These strategies prevent the tragic consequence of missing data.

Although it is not frequently practiced, we find it useful and important to evaluate the predictive performance of the final logistic model. To this end, we make use of ROC (receiver operating characteristic) curves (see, e.g., Hanley, 1989). We know that we cannot always make perfect classification or prediction for the outcome of interest. For this reason, we want to make as few mistakes as possible. Two kinds of mistakes can occur when we predict an ill-conditioned outcome as normal or a normal condition as abnormal. To distinguish them, statisticians refer these mistakes to as type I and type II errors, respectively. In medical-decision making, they are called false-negative and false-positive diagnoses, respectively. In reasonable settings, these errors oppose each other. That is, reducing the rate of one type of error elevates the rate of the other type of error. ROC curves reflect both rates and quantify the accuracy of the prediction through a graphical presentation.

For subject i, we estimate her risk [probability] of having preterm delivery by

$$p = \hat{\theta}_i = \frac{\exp(-2.344 - 0.076 x_{i6} + 0.699 z_{i6} + 0.115 x_{i,11} + 1.539 z_{i,10})}{1 + \exp(-2.344 - 0.076 x_{i6} + 0.699 z_{i6} + 0.115 x_{i,11} + 1.539 z_{i,10})}, \quad (3.3)$$

$i = 1, \ldots, 3861$, using the estimates in Table 3.3. For any risk threshold r ($0 \leq r \leq 1$), we calculate the empirical true and false positive probabilities respectively as

$$TPP = \frac{\text{the number of preterm deliveries for which } \hat{\theta}_i > r}{\text{the total number of preterm deliveries}}$$

and

$$FPP = \frac{\text{the number of term deliveries for which } \hat{\theta}_i > r}{\text{the total number of term deliveries}}.$$

As r varies continuously, the trace of (TPP, FPP) constitutes the ROC curve as shown in Figure 3.1. In the medical literature, the true positive and negative probabilities are commonly referred to as sensitivity and specificity.

Figure 3.1 indicates that the final logistic regression model improves the predictive precision over a random prediction model. The latter predicts the risk of 1 and 0 by tossing a fair coin. The ROC curve for this random prediction is featured by the dotted straight line. It is evident from Figure 3.1 that a great deal of variation is not explained and hence that further improvement should be sought.

Note also that the ROC curve is drawn from the resubstitution estimate of the risk, which tends to be optimistic in the sense that the ROC curve may have an upward-biased area. The reason is as follows. The prediction in (3.3) was derived to "maximize" the area under the ROC curve based on the Yale Pregnancy Outcome Study data. If we conduct another similar, independent study, which we call a validation study, it is almost sure that we will end up with an optimal prediction that differs from equation (3.3), although the difference may not be large. The other side of the coin is that if we make predictions for the subjects in the validation study from equation (3.3), the quality of the prediction is usually downgraded as compared to the prediction made for the original Yale Pregnancy Outcome Study. In

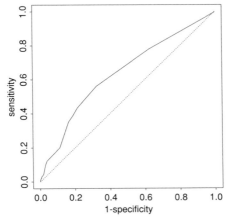

FIGURE 3.1. ROC curve for the final logistic regression model

some applications, validation studies are available, e.g., Goldman et al. (1982, 1996). In most cases, investigators have only one set of data. To assess the quality of the prediction, certain sample reuse techniques such as the cross-validation procedure are warranted (e.g., Efron, 1983). The cross-validation procedure will be heavily used in this book, specifically in Chapters 4, and 8–11. The basic idea is that we build our models using part of the available data and reserve the left-out observations to validate the selected models. This is a way to create an artificial validation study at the cost of reducing the sample size for estimating a model. The simplest strategy is to cut the entire sample into two pieces of equal size. While one piece is used to build a model, the other piece tests the model. It is a sample reuse mechanism because we can alternate the roles for the two pieces of sample.

4
Classification Trees for a Binary Response

In this chapter we discuss the technical aspect of the recursive partitioning technique, following the brief introduction from Chapter 2. This chapter, particularly the less technical parts of it, is helpful for understanding the methodological and theoretical aspects of recursive partitioning as well as for efficiently and correctly using the computer software. For clarity, we concentrate on the simplest case—a binary response. However, the basic framework of recursive partitioning is established here.

4.1 Node Impurity

Since a tree consists of nodes, the property of the tree depends on that of the nodes. We introduced the entropy impurity in (2.1) and (2.2) as one measure for assessing the node homogeneity. As described by Breiman et al. (1984), there are also other choices of impurity functions. Here, we present a general definition of node impurity.

As we are presently concerned with a binary outcome, the impurity of a node τ is defined as a nonnegative function of the probability, $P\{Y=1|\tau\}$, which is the prevalence rate of diseased (or ill-conditioned) subjects in the group represented by node τ. Intuitively, the least impure node should have only one class of the outcome (i.e., $P\{Y=1|\tau\} = 0$ or 1), and its impurity is zero. For instance, all terminal nodes in Figure 2.1 are pure. On the other hand, node τ is most impure when $P\{Y=1|\tau\} = \frac{1}{2}$. That is, if we take a subject from node τ, it is equally likely that this subject

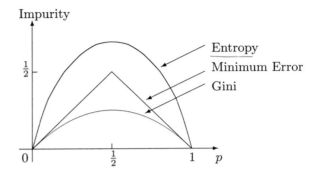

FIGURE 4.1. Impurity functions

is an ill-conditioned or a normal subject. In general, the impurity function has a concave shape (see Figure 4.1) and can be formally defined as

$$i(\tau) = \phi(I\!P\{Y = 1 \,|\, \tau\}), \qquad (4.1)$$

where the function ϕ has the properties (i) $\phi \geq 0$ and (ii) for any $p \in (0,1)$, $\phi(p) = \phi(1-p)$ and $\phi(0) = \phi(1) < \phi(p)$.

Common choices of ϕ include

$$\begin{align}
\text{(i)} \quad & \phi(p) = \min(p, 1-p), & (4.2) \\
\text{(ii)} \quad & \phi(p) = -p\log(p) - (1-p)\log(1-p), & (4.3) \\
\text{(iii)} \quad & \phi(p) = p(1-p), & (4.4)
\end{align}$$

where $0\log 0 = 0$. They are illustrated by Figure 4.1. In the context of discriminating a binary class, Devroye et al. (1996, p. 29) call these ϕ's the F-errors. In particular, (4.2) is the Bayes error, i.e., the minimum error; (4.3) is the entropy function; and (4.4) is half of the asymptotic nearest neighbor error, or Gini index. The Bayes error is rarely used in practice due to some undesirable properties as explained by Breiman et al. (1984, p. 99). The Gini criterion also has some problems, as will be pointed out at the end of this section. Hence, from now on the impurity refers to the entropy criterion unless stated otherwise.

The computation of impurity is simple when the prevalence rate $I\!P\{Y = 1 \,|\, \tau\}$ in node τ is available. In many applications such as prospective studies, this prevalence rate can be estimated empirically from the data. At other times, additional prior information may be required to estimate the prevalence rate. For example, let us consider a case-control study with, say, 100 controls and 100 cases. We need to know or guess a priori the prevalence rate for the disease of interest among the underlying population from which the 200 study subjects are selected and to which we would generalize our conclusions. As an example, suppose that the population prevalence is 0.004. That is, there are four cases per 1,000 subjects randomly selected from the population. Then, using Bayes' theorem, the prevalence rate within a node τ is

$$\mathbb{P}\{Y=1\,|\,\tau\} \;=\; \frac{\mathbb{P}\{Y=1,\tau\}}{\mathbb{P}\{\tau\}}$$

$$=\; \frac{\mathbb{P}\{Y=1\}\mathbb{P}\{\tau\,|\,Y=1\}}{\mathbb{P}\{Y=1\}\mathbb{P}\{\tau\,|\,Y=1\}+\mathbb{P}\{Y=0\}\mathbb{P}\{\tau\,|\,Y=0\}},$$

where, marginally, $\mathbb{P}\{Y=1\} = 1 - \mathbb{P}\{Y=0\} = 0.004$. The conditional probabilities $\mathbb{P}\{\tau\,|\,Y=1\}$ and $\mathbb{P}\{\tau\,|\,Y=0\}$ can be estimated from the data. The former is the conditional probability for a random subject to fall into node τ given that the subject's response is 1. The latter conditional probability has a similar interpretation. Suppose that 30 of the 100 cases and 50 of the 100 controls fall into node τ. Then, $\mathbb{P}\{\tau\,|\,Y=1\} = 30/100 = 0.3$ and $\mathbb{P}\{\tau\,|\,Y=0\} = 50/100 = 0.5$. Putting together these figures, we obtain

$$\mathbb{P}\{Y=1\,|\,\tau\} = \frac{0.004*0.3}{0.004*0.3+0.996*0.5} = 0.0024.$$

The criterion first defined in (2.1) and again in (4.3) has another interpretation. This different view is helpful in generalizing the tree-based methods for various purposes. Suppose that Y in node τ_L follows a binomial distribution with a frequency of θ, namely,

$$\mathbb{P}\{Y=1\,|\,\tau_L\} = \theta.$$

Then, the log-likelihood function from the n_1. observations in node τ_L is

$$n_{11}\log(\theta) + n_{12}\log(1-\theta).$$

The maximum of this log-likelihood function is

$$n_{11}\log\left(\frac{n_{11}}{n_1.}\right) + n_{12}\log\left(\frac{n_{12}}{n_1.}\right),$$

which is proportional to (2.1). In light of this fact, many node-splitting criteria originate from the maximum of certain likelihood functions. The importance of this observation will be appreciated in Chapters 8 and 10.

So far, we only made use of an impurity function for node splitting. There are also alternative approaches. In particular, it is noteworthy to mention the twoing rule (Breiman et al., 1984, p. 38) that uses a different measure for the goodness of a split as follows:

$$\frac{\mathbb{P}\{\tau_L\}\mathbb{P}\{\tau_R\}}{4}\left[\sum_{j=0,1}|\mathbb{P}\{Y=j|\tau_L\}-\mathbb{P}\{Y=j|\tau_R\}|\right]^2.$$

For a binary response, this twoing rule coincides with the use of the Gini index. It has been observed that this rule has an undesirable end-cut preference problem (Morgan and Messenger, 1973 and Breiman et al., 1984,

Ch. 11): It gives preference to the splits that result in two daughter nodes of extremely unbalanced sizes. To resolve this problem, a modification, called the delta splitting rule, has been adopted in both the THAID (Messenger and Mandell, 1972 and Morgan and Messenger, 1973) and CART (Breiman et al., 1984) programs. Other split functions may also suffer from this problem, but our observations seem to indicate that the Gini index is more problematic.

4.2 Determination of Terminal Nodes

Recall that the objective of recursive partitioning is to extract homogeneous subgroups of the study sample. Whether we have achieved this objective depends on whether the terminal nodes are indeed homogeneous. In other words, the quality of a tree is merely the quality of its terminal nodes. Hence, for a tree T we define

$$R(T) = \sum_{\tau \in \tilde{T}} I\!P\{\tau\}r(\tau), \qquad (4.5)$$

where $\tilde{T}$ is the set of terminal nodes of T and $r(\tau)$ measures a certain quality of node τ, as will be specified in the following two sections. Broadly speaking, $r(\tau)$ is similar to the sum of the squared residuals in the linear regression. The purpose of pruning is to select the best subtree, T^*, of an initially saturated tree, T_0, such that $R(T)$ is minimized. We will explain how to determine terminal nodes, or equivalently, the subtree T^*, in the following four subsections. Readers who are less interested in the methodological development may skip them.

4.2.1 Misclassification Cost

We have several issues to take care of. First, we need to define $r(\tau)$ from which we establish the tree quality, $R(T)$. Then, we discuss how to estimate $R(T)$ and how to use it in pruning a tree.

The node impurity is an obvious candidate for $r(\tau)$. In the present context, however, $r(\tau)$ is commonly chosen as the misclassification cost, because we are focused on *classifying* the binary outcome. By the same token, one would wonder why we do not partition the node by minimizing the misclassification cost in the first place. We defer the answer to the end of this section. Nevertheless, in Chapters 8 and 10 we see that $r(\tau)$ and the splitting criterion are sometimes based on the same measure.

In many applications, the tree-based method is used for the purpose of prediction. That is, given the characteristics of a subject, we must predict the outcome of this subject before we know the outcome. For example, in the study of Goldman et al. (1982), physicians in emergency rooms must predict whether a patient with chest pain suffers from a serious heart disease based on the information available within a few hours of admission. To this end, we first classify a node τ to either class 0 (normal) or 1 (abnormal), and we predict the outcome of an individual based on the membership of the node to which the individual belongs. Unfortunately, we always make mistakes in such a classification, because some of the normal subjects will be predicted as diseased and vice versa. For instance, Figure 3.1 pinpoints the predictive performance of a logistic regression model in terms of these false positive errors and false negative errors. In any case, to weigh these mistakes, we need to assign misclassification costs.

Let us take the root node in Figure 2.2(b). In this root node, there are 205 preterm and 3,656 term deliveries. If we assign class 1 for the root node, 3,656 normal subjects are misclassified. In this case, we would wrongly predict normal subjects to be abnormal, and false positive errors occur. On the other hand, we misclassify the 205 abnormal subjects if the root node is assigned class 0. These are false negative errors. If what matters is the count of the false positive and the false negative errors, we would assign class 0 for the root node, because we then make fewer mistakes. This naive classification, however, fails to take into account the seriousness of the mistakes. For example, when we classify a term delivery as preterm, the baby may receive "unnecessary" special care. But if a preterm baby is thought to be in term, the baby may not get needed care. Sometimes, a mistake could be fatal, such as a false negative diagnosis of heart failure. In most applications, the false negative errors are more serious than the false positive errors. Consequently, we cannot simply count the errors. The two kinds of mistakes must be weighted.

Let $c(i|j)$ be a unit misclassification cost that a class j subject is classified as a class i subject. When $i = j$, we have the correct classification and the cost should naturally be zero, i.e., $c(i|i) = 0$. Since i and j take only the values of 0 or 1, without loss of generality we can set $c(1|0) = 1$. In other words, one false positive error counts as one. The clinicians and the statisticians need to work together to gauge the relative cost of $c(0|1)$. This is a subjective and difficult, but important, decision. Later, in Section 4.5 we will introduce an alternative pruning procedure that avoids this decision.

Here, for the purpose of illustration, we take a range of values between 1 and 18 for $c(0|1)$. For the reasons cited above, we usually assume that $c(0|1) \geq c(1|0)$. The upper bound 18 is based on the fact that $3656 : 205 = 17.8 : 1$. Note that 3656 and 205 are the numbers of term and preterm deliveries in the root node, respectively. Table 4.1 reports the misclassification costs for the five nodes in Figure 2.2(b) when these nodes are assumed either as class 0 or as class 1.

For example, when $c(0|1) = 10$, it means that one false negative error counts as many as ten false positive ones. We know that the cost is 3656 if the root node is assigned class 1. It becomes $225 \times 10 = 2250$ if the root node is assigned class 0. Therefore, the root node should be assigned class

34   4. Classification Trees for a Binary Response

TABLE 4.1. Misclassification Costs

	Assumed Class	Node number				
		1	2	3	4	5
$c(0\|1)$	1	3656	640	3016	187	453
1	0	205	70	135	11	59
10	0	2050	700	1350	110	590
18	0	3690	1260	2430	198	1062

0 for $2250 < 3656$. In other words, the class membership of 0 or 1 for a node depends on whether or not the cost of the false positive errors is lower than that of the false negative errors. Formally, node τ is assigned class j if

$$\sum_i [c(j|i) I\!P\{Y = i | \tau\}] \leq \sum_i [c(1-j|i) I\!P\{Y = i | \tau\}]. \quad (4.6)$$

Denote the left-hand side of (4.6) by $r(\tau)$, which is the expected cost resulting from any subject within the node. This cost is usually referred to as the within-node misclassification cost. It appears less confusing, however, to call it the conditional misclassification cost. Multiplying $r(\tau)$ by $I\!P\{\tau\}$, we have the unconditional misclassification cost of the node, $R(\tau) = I\!P\{\tau\}r(\tau)$. In the following discussions, the misclassification cost of a node implies the unconditional definition, and the within-node misclassification cost means the conditional one.

Earlier in this section, we mentioned the possibility of using $r(\tau)$ to split nodes. This proves to be inconvenient in the present case, because it is usually difficult to assign the cost function before any tree is grown. As a matter of fact, the assignment can still be challenging even when a tree profile is given. Moreover, there is abundant empirical evidence that the use of an impurity function such as the entropy generally leads to useful trees with reasonable sample sizes. We refer to Breiman et al. (1984) for some examples.

Having defined the misclassification cost for a node and hence a tree, we face the issue of estimating it. In this section, we take $c(0|1) = 10$, for example. The process is the same with regard to other choices of $c(0|1)$. According to Table 4.1, we can estimate the misclassification costs for nodes 1 to 5 in Figure 2.2(b). As reported in Table 4.2, these estimates are called resubstitution estimates of the misclassification cost.

Let $R^s(\tau)$ denote the resubstitution estimate of the misclassification cost for node τ. Unfortunately, the resubstitution estimates generally underestimate the cost in the following sense. If we have an independent data set, we can assign the new subjects to various nodes of the tree and calculate the cost based on these new subjects. This cost tends to be higher than the resubstitution estimate, because the split criteria are somehow related to the cost, and as a result, the resubstitution estimate of misclassification

4.2 Determination of Terminal Nodes

TABLE 4.2. Resubstitution Estimates of Misclassification Costs (unit cost: $c(0|1) = 10$)

Node number	Node class	Weight $I\!P\{\tau\}$	×	Within-node cost $r(\tau)$	Cost $R^s(\tau)$
1	0	$\frac{3861}{3861}$		$\frac{10*205}{3861}$	$\frac{2050}{3861} = 0.531$
2	1	$\frac{710}{3861}$		$\frac{1*640}{710}$	$\frac{640}{3861} = 0.166$
3	0	$\frac{3151}{3861}$		$\frac{10*135}{3151}$	$\frac{1350}{3861} = 0.35$
4	0	$\frac{198}{3861}$		$\frac{10*11}{198}$	$\frac{110}{3861} = 0.028$
5	1	$\frac{506}{3861}$		$\frac{1*453}{506}$	$\frac{453}{3861} = 0.117$

(handwritten annotation: terminal nodes — indicating rows 3, 4, 5)

cost is usually over optimistic. In some applications, such an independent data set, called a test sample or validation set, is available; see, e.g., Goldman et al. (1982, 1996). To obtain unbiased cost estimates, sample reuse procedures such as cross-validation are warranted.

4.2.2 Cost Complexity

Although the concept of misclassification cost has its own merit, a major use of it in the tree context is to select a "right-sized" subtree, namely, to determine the terminal nodes. For example, in Figure 2.2, panel (a) represents a subtree of the tree in panel (b). Because a tree (or subtree) gives an integrated picture of nodes, we concentrate here on how to estimate the misclassification cost for a tree. This motivation leads to a very critical concept in the tree methodology: tree cost-complexity. It is defined as

$$R_\alpha(\mathcal{T}) = R(\mathcal{T}) + \alpha|\tilde{\mathcal{T}}|, \tag{4.7}$$

where α (≥ 0) is the complexity parameter and $|\tilde{\mathcal{T}}|$ is the number of terminal nodes in $\mathcal{T}$. Here, the tree complexity is really another term for the tree size. $|\tilde{\mathcal{T}}|$ is used as a measure of tree complexity, because the total number of nodes in tree $\mathcal{T}$ is twice the number of its terminal nodes minus 1, i.e., $|\mathcal{T}| = 2|\tilde{\mathcal{T}}| - 1$. The difference between $R_\alpha(\mathcal{T})$ and $R(\mathcal{T})$ as a measure of tree quality resides in that $R_\alpha(\mathcal{T})$ penalizes a big tree.

For any tree with over, say, 20 nodes, many subtrees are possible, and the combinatorics involved are usually complicated. The use of tree cost-complexity allows us to construct a sequence of nested "essential" subtrees from any given tree $\mathcal{T}$ so that we can examine the properties of these subtrees and make a selection from them.

We earlier discarded the idea of using the resubstitution approach to estimate the node misclassification cost. The resubstitution approach, however, plays a different, useful, role in evaluating the cost-complexity. Let us take another look at the five-node tree, denoted by $\mathcal{T}_0$, in Figure 2.2(b). Using the resubstitution estimates in Table 4.2, the cost for $\mathcal{T}_0$ is $0.350 + 0.028 +$

$0.117 = 0.495$ and its complexity is 3. Thus, its cost-complexity is $0.495+3\alpha$ for a given complexity parameter α. The question is, Is there a subtree of T_0 that has a smaller cost-complexity? The following fact is critical to the answer to this question.

Theorem 4.1 (Breiman et al., 1984, Section 3.3) *For any value of the complexity parameter α, there is a unique smallest subtree of T_0 that minimizes the cost-complexity.*

This theorem ensures that we cannot have two subtrees of the smallest size and of the same cost-complexity. We call this smallest subtree the optimal subtree with respect to the complexity parameter. For example, when $\alpha = 0$, the optimal subtree is T_0 itself. Why? Note that T_0 has two additional subtrees. One, denoted by T_1, is plotted in Figure 2.2(a) and its cost-complexity is $0.166 + 0.350 + 0 * 2 = 0.516$. The other subtree, call it T_2, contains only the root node, and its cost-complexity is $0.531 + 0 * 1 = 0.531$. We see that both 0.516 and 0.531 are greater than 0.495. In general, however, the optimal subtree corresponding to $\alpha = 0$ may not be the initial tree.

We can always choose α large enough that the corresponding optimal subtree is the single-node tree. In fact, when $\alpha \geq 0.018$, T_2 (the root node tree) becomes the optimal subtree, because

$$R_{0.018}(T_2) = 0.531 + 0.018 * 1 = 0.495 + 0.018 * 3 = R_{0.018}(T_0)$$

and

$$R_{0.018}(T_2) = 0.531 + 0.018 * 1 < 0.516 + 0.018 * 2 = R_{0.018}(T_1).$$

Although $R_{0.018}(T_2) = R_{0.018}(T_0)$, T_2 is the optimal subtree, because it is smaller than T_0. This calculation confirms the theorem that we do not have two subtrees of the smallest size and of the same cost-complexity.

It is interesting to point out that T_1 is not an optimal subtree for any α. This is because T_0 is the optimal subtree for any $\alpha \in [0, 0.018)$ and T_2 is the optimal subtree when $\alpha \in [0.018, \infty)$. Two observations are noteworthy. First, not all subtrees are optimal with respect to a complexity parameter. This is important, because we cannot afford to consider all subtrees. We regard such subtrees as nonessential. Second, although the complexity parameter takes a continuous range of values, we have only a finite number of subtrees. Consequently, an optimal subtree is optimal for an interval range of the complexity parameter, and the number of such intervals has to be finite. For example, our tree T_0 gives rise to two intervals.

It remains to find the limits of these intervals, or the thresholds of α and to make use of the corresponding optimal subtrees. These issues will be addressed in Section 4.2.3.

4.2.3 Nested Optimal Subtrees*

To have a better picture, we use an expanded tree structure as displayed in Figure 4.2, in which the nodes are numbered from 1 to 9. Note that each internal node has a number of offspring terminal nodes. We derive the first positive threshold parameter, α_1, for this tree by comparing the resubstitution misclassification cost of an internal node to the sum of the resubstitution misclassification costs of its offspring terminal nodes. The latter is denoted by $R^s(\tilde{T}_\tau)$ for a node τ. Here, T_τ may be viewed as a subtree rooted at node τ, and $\tilde{T}_\tau$ contains the terminal nodes of T_τ, i.e., the offspring terminal nodes of node τ in the larger tree.

Table 4.3 presents $R^s(\tau)$, $R^s(\tilde{T}_\tau)$, and $|\tilde{T}_\tau|$ in columns 2 to 4, respectively. This information is vital to the comparison of the cost-complexity of a node with those of its offspring terminal nodes. For example, the cost of node 3 per se is $R^s(3) = 1350/3861 = 0.350$. It is the ancestor of terminal nodes 7, 8, and 9. The units of misclassification cost within these three terminal nodes are respectively 154, 25, and 1120. Hence, $R^s(\tilde{T}_3) = (154 + 25 + 1120)/3861 = 0.336$. Thus, the difference between $R^s(3)$ and $R^s(\tilde{T}_3)$ is $0.350 - 0.336 = 0.014$. On the other hand, the difference in complexity between node 3 alone and its three offspring terminal nodes is $3 - 1 = 2$. On average, an additional terminal node reduces the cost by $0.014/2 = 0.007$, as given in the last column of Table 4.3.

The question is, What happens if an internal node becomes a terminal node? In other words, what is the consequence of pruning off all offspring nodes of an internal node? For instance, if we cut the offspring nodes of the root node, we have the root-node tree whose cost-complexity is $0.531 + \alpha$. For it to have the same cost-complexity as the initial nine-node tree, we need $0.481 + 5\alpha = 0.531 + \alpha$, giving $\alpha = 0.013$. We can also find out the consequence of changing node 2 to a terminal node. Then, the initial nine-node tree is compared with a seven-node subtree, consisting of nodes 1 to 3, and 6 to 9. For the new subtree to have the same cost-complexity as the initial tree, we find $\alpha = 0.021$. In fact, for any internal node, $\tau \notin \tilde{T}$, the value of α is precisely

$$\frac{R^s(\tau) - R^s(\tilde{T}_\tau)}{|\tilde{T}_\tau| - 1}.$$

The first positive threshold parameter, α_1, is the smallest α over the $|\tilde{T}| - 1$ internal nodes. According to Table 4.3, $\alpha_1 = 0.007$ for the present example.

Using α_1 we change an internal node τ to a terminal node when

$$R^s(\tau) + \alpha_1 \leq R^s(\tilde{T}_\tau) + \alpha_1|\tilde{T}_\tau|$$

until this is not possible. This pruning process results in the optimal subtree corresponding to α_1. In fact, this first threshold yields the tree presented in Figure 2.2(b).

After pruning the tree using the first threshold, we seek the second threshold complexity parameter, α_2, in the same way as the first one except

38   4. Classification Trees for a Binary Response

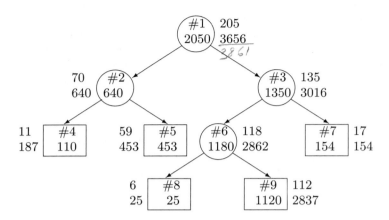

FIGURE 4.2. Construction of nested optimal trees. Inside each node are the node number (top) and the units of the misclassification cost (bottom). Next to the node are the number of abnormal (top) and normal (bottom) subjects in the node.

TABLE 4.3. Cost Complexity

Node	$R^s(\tau)$	$R^s(\tilde{\mathcal{T}}_\tau)$	$|\tilde{\mathcal{T}}_\tau|$	α
9	0.290	0.290	1	
8	0.006	0.006	1	
7	0.040	0.040	1	
6	0.306	0.296	2	0.010
5	0.117	0.117	1	
4	0.028	0.028	1	
3	0.350	0.336	3	0.007
2	0.166	0.145	2	0.021
1	0.531	0.481	5	0.013
		Minimum		0.007

that the once pruned subtree in Figure 2.4(b) plays the role of an initial tree. We knew from our previous discussion that $\alpha_2 = 0.018$ and its optimal subtree is the root-node tree. No more thresholds need to be found from here, because the root-node tree is the smallest one.

In general, suppose that we end up with m thresholds,

$$0 < \alpha_1 < \alpha_2 < \cdots < \alpha_m, \tag{4.8}$$

and let $\alpha_0 = 0$. The threshold α_k ($k = 0, \ldots, m$) must increase by construction. Also, let the corresponding optimal subtrees be

$$\mathcal{T}_{\alpha_0} \supset \mathcal{T}_{\alpha_1} \supset \mathcal{T}_{\alpha_2} \supset \cdots \supset \mathcal{T}_{\alpha_m}, \tag{4.9}$$

where $\mathcal{T}_{\alpha_1} \supset \mathcal{T}_{\alpha_2}$ means that $\mathcal{T}_{\alpha_2}$ is a subtree of $\mathcal{T}_{\alpha_1}$. In particular, $\mathcal{T}_{\alpha_m}$ is the root-node subtree. These are so-called nested optimal subtrees. The final subtree will be selected from among them.

The construction of the nested optimal subtrees proves the following useful result:

Theorem 4.2 *If $\alpha_1 > \alpha_2$, the optimal subtree corresponding to α_1 is a subtree of the optimal subtree corresponding to α_2.*

To pave the road for the final selection, what we need is a good estimate of $R(\mathcal{T}_{\alpha_k})$ ($k = 0, 1, \ldots, m$), namely, the misclassification costs of the subtrees. We will select the one with the smallest misclassification cost.

When a test sample is available, estimating $R(\mathcal{T})$ for any subtree $\mathcal{T}$ is straightforward, because we only need to apply the subtrees to the test sample. Difficulty arises when we do not have a test sample. The cross-validation process is generally used by creating artificial test samples. The idea will be described shortly.

Before describing the cross-validation process, we may find it helpful to recall what we have achieved so far. Beginning with a learning sample, we can construct a large tree by recursively splitting the nodes. From this large tree, we then compute a sequence of complexity parameters $\{\alpha_k\}_0^m$ and their corresponding optimal subtrees $\{\mathcal{T}_{\alpha_k}\}_0^m$.

The first step of cross-validation is to divide the entire study sample into a number of pieces, usually 5, 10, or 25 corresponding to 5-, 10-, or 25-fold cross-validation, respectively. Here, let us randomly divide the 3,861 women in the Yale Pregnancy Outcome Study into 5 groups: 1 to 5. Group 1 has 773 women and each of the rest contains 772 women. Let $\mathcal{L}_{(-i)}$ be the sample set including all but those subjects in group i, $i = 1, \ldots, 5$.

Using the 3,088 women in $\mathcal{L}_{(-1)}$, we can surely produce another large tree, say $\mathcal{T}_{(-1)}$, in the same way as we did using all 3,861 women. Take each α_k from the sequence of complexity parameters as has already been derived above and obtain the optimal subtree, $\mathcal{T}_{(-1),k}$, of $\mathcal{T}_{(-1)}$ corresponding to α_k. Then, we would have a sequence of the optimal subtrees of $\mathcal{T}_{(-1)}$, i.e.,

$\{\mathcal{T}_{(-1),k}\}_0^m$. Using group 1 as a test sample relative to $\mathcal{L}_{(-1)}$, we have an unbiased estimate, $R^{ts}(\mathcal{T}_{(-1),k})$, of $R(\mathcal{T}_{(-1),k})$. Because $\mathcal{T}_{(-1),k}$ is related to $\mathcal{T}_{\alpha_k}$ through the same α_k, $R^{ts}(\mathcal{T}_{(-1),k})$ can be regarded as a cross-validation estimate of $R(\mathcal{T}_{\alpha_k})$. Likewise, using $\mathcal{L}_{(-i)}$ as the learning sample and the data in group i as the test sample, we also have $R^{ts}(\mathcal{T}_{(-i),k})$, $(i = 2, \ldots, 5)$ as the cross-validation estimate of $R(\mathcal{T}_{\alpha_k})$. Thus, the final cross-validation estimate, $R^{cv}(\mathcal{T}_{\alpha_k})$, of $R(\mathcal{T}_{\alpha_k})$ follows from averaging $R^{ts}(\mathcal{T}_{(-i),k})$ over $i = 1, \ldots, 5$.

The subtree corresponding to the smallest R^{cv} is obviously desirable. As we see in Section 4.4, the cross-validation estimates generally have substantial variabilities. Bearing in mind the uncertainty of the estimation process and the desire of constructing a parsimonious tree structure, Breiman et al. (1984) proposed a revised strategy to select the final tree, which takes into account the standard errors of the cross-validation estimates. Let SE_k be the standard error for $R^{cv}(\mathcal{T}_{\alpha_k})$. We discuss how to derive SE_k in Section 4.3. Suppose that $R^{cv}(\mathcal{T}_{\alpha_{k^*}})$ is the smallest among all $R^{cv}(\mathcal{T}_{\alpha_k})$'s. The revised selection rule selects the smallest subtree whose cross-validation estimate is within a prespecified range of $R^{cv}(\mathcal{T}_{\alpha_{k^*}})$, which is usually defined by one unit of SE_{k^*}. This is the so-called 1-SE rule. Empirical evidence suggests that the tree selected with the 1-SE rule is more often than not superior to the one selected with 0-SE rule (namely, the tree with the minimal R^{cv}). We will revisit the Yale Pregnancy Outcome Study in Section 4.4 and present the numerical details of the entire tree-growing and pruning steps including the cross-validation procedure.

4.3 The Standard Error of R^{cv*}

It is always important to gauge the uncertainty of the statistical estimates. Given the complexity of the recursive partitioning procedure, it is intricate and perhaps even impossible to derive the standard error for the cross-validation estimate of the tree misclassification cost. Many factors contribute to this complication: We make no distributional assumptions regarding the response, and the tree is determined by a forward stepwise growing procedure followed by a nested, bottom-up pruning step. The tree pruning is particularly complicated and makes analytic derivations prohibitive. What follows is the heuristic argument given by Breiman et al. (1984, Section 11.5). For more theoretically oriented readers, this heuristic argument may serve as a starting point.

Recall that every subject in the entire study sample was used once as a testing subject and was assigned a class membership $m + 1$ times through the sequence of $m + 1$ subtrees built upon the corresponding learning sample. Let $C_{i,k}$ be the misclassification cost incurred for the ith subject while it was a testing subject and the classification rule was based on the kth subtree, $i = 1, \ldots, n$, $k = 0, 1, \ldots, m$. Then,

$$R^{cv}(\mathcal{T}_{\alpha_k}) = \sum_{j=0,1} \mathbb{P}\{Y = j\} \bar{C}_{k|j}, \qquad (4.10)$$

where $\bar{C}_{k|j}$ is the average of $C_{i,k}$ over the set S_j of the subjects whose response is j (i.e., $Y = j$). Namely,

$$\bar{C}_{k|j} = \frac{1}{n_j} \sum_{i \in S_j} C_{i,k}, \qquad (4.11)$$

where n_j is the number of subjects in S_j. We know that $C_{i,k}$'s are likely to be correlated with each other, because $C_{i,k}$ is the cost from the same subject (the ith one) while the subtree (the kth one) varies. For convenience, however, they are treated as if they were not correlated. Then, the sample variance of each $\bar{C}_{k|j}$ is

$$\frac{1}{n_j^2} \left(\sum_{i \in S_j} C_{i,k}^2 - n_j \bar{C}_{k|j}^2 \right),$$

and it follows from (4.10) and (4.11) that the heuristic standard error for $R^{cv}(\mathcal{T}_{\alpha_k})$ is given by

$$\mathrm{SE}_k = \left\{ \sum_{j=0,1} \left(\frac{\mathbb{P}\{Y = j\}}{n_j} \right)^2 \left(\sum_{i \in S_j} C_{i,k}^2 - n_j \bar{C}_{k|j}^2 \right) \right\}^{1/2}. \qquad (4.12)$$

4.4 Tree-Based Analysis of the Yale Pregnancy Outcome Study

In this section we apply the recursive partitioning technique to the data from the Yale Pregnancy Outcome Study. Figure 4.3 is the sketch of a large tree with 53 nodes. This large tree produces a sequence of 11 nested optimal subtrees corresponding to 11 complexity parameters, $\{\alpha_k\}_0^{10}$. Again, we choose $C(0|1) = 10$. In Figure 4.3, these complexity parameters are placed at the nodes that could become terminal nodes for the given parameters. We can see the gradual change of the tree structure as we increase the complexity parameter.

Using the cross-validation procedure, we estimated the misclassification costs for the 11 optimal subtrees and then calculated their standard errors via (4.12). We used 5- and 10-fold each once, and the numerical results are reported in Figure 4.4. The variation between the estimates from 5- and 10-fold cross-validations seems to suggest that the standard error given in

42   4. Classification Trees for a Binary Response

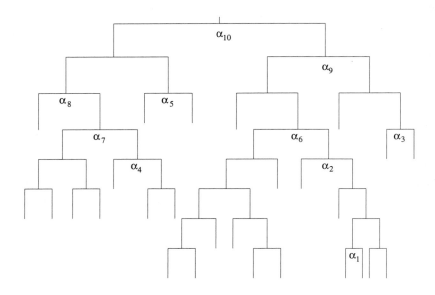

FIGURE 4.3. An initial large tree indexed by a sequence of complexity parameters

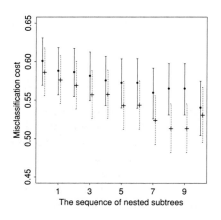

FIGURE 4.4. Cross-validation estimates of misclassification cost for a sequence of nested optimal trees. 5- and 10-fold estimates are respectively indicated by • and +. Also plotted along the estimates are the intervals of length of two SE's (1 SE along each direction).

(4.12) may be slightly underestimated. A more thorough examination may be done by repeating the cross-validation procedure a number of times and computing the empirical estimates of standard error.

Figure 4.4 indicates that the 1-SE rule selects the root-node subtree. The interpretation is that the risk factors considered here may not have enough predictive power to stand out and pass the cross-validation. This statement is obviously relative to the selected unit cost $C(0|1) = 10$. For instance, when we used $C(0|1) = 18$ and performed a 5-fold cross-validation, the final tree had a similar structure to the one presented in Figure 4.2 except that node 2 should be a terminal node. When the purpose of the analysis is exploratory, we may prune a tree using alternative approaches. See the next section for the details.

4.5 An Alternative Pruning Approach

We see from the discussion in Section 4.4 that the choice of the penalty for a false negative error, $C(0|1) = 10$, is vital to the selection of the final tree structure. It must be appropriately chosen and justified if classifying subjects is the primary aim of the analysis. In many secondary analyses, however, the purpose is mainly to explore the data structure and to generate hypotheses. See, e.g., Zhang and Bracken (1995, 1996). Thus, it would be convenient to proceed with the analysis without assigning the unit of misclassification cost. In later chapters (8 and 10), when we deal with responses of a more complicated nature, it would be even harder or infeasible to adopt the idea of assigning misclassification costs. Moreover, as discussed by Zhang et al. (1996), the premise under which the cross-validation procedure is performed may not hold in some practices, because we may grow and prune trees manually. Furthermore, in some data for which variables may be grouped broadly as genetic and environmental, it may be interesting to have genetic factors appear before the environmental ones during the recursive partitioning. In other situations, information may be collected sequentially, and it can be important to partition the data using the variables that are readily available. Finally, ad hoc tree "repairs" may be desirable on a case-by-case basis. This involves changing the splitting variables and splitting levels so that the tree structure is easier to interpret in a clinical sense. To summarize, a tree structure resulting from an automatic procedure is not necessarily what we would like to have. Sometimes, there may also be a methodological and/or practical incentive to seek alternative backward pruning procedures. Next, we describe one such procedure in the spirit of the proposal suggested by Segal (1988) for survival trees (see Chapter 8).

After the large tree $\mathcal{T}$ is grown, assign a statistic S_τ to each internal node τ from the bottom up. We shall return to the detail of this assignment later.

Then, we align these statistics in increasing order as
$$S_{\tau_1} \leq S_{\tau_2} \leq \cdots \leq S_{\tau_{|\tilde{T}|-1}}.$$
Select a threshold level and change an internal node to a terminal one if its statistic is less than the threshold level. Two approaches are available for choosing the threshold. A simple one is to take a threshold corresponding to a specified significance level, say 0.05.

The second approach constructs a sequence of nested subtrees in the spirit of Section 4.2.3, and the threshold merges as a result of reviewing these nested subtrees. The nested subtrees are produced as follows: Locate the smallest S_τ over all internal nodes and prune the offspring of the highest node(s) that reaches this minimum. What remains is the first subtree. Repeat the same process again and again until the subtree contains the root node only. As the process continues, a sequence of nested subtrees, $T_1, \ldots, T_m$, will be produced. To select a threshold value, we make a plot of $\min_{\tau \in T_i - \tilde{T}_i} S_\tau$ versus $|\tilde{T}_i|$, i.e., the minimal statistic of a subtree against its size. Then, we look for a possible "kink" in this plot where the pattern changes. Although this seems subjective, it offers us an opportunity to apply our clinical knowledge together with the purely statistical information to determine the final tree structure.

Let us use the large tree in Figure 4.3 and see what happens when this alternative pruning approach is applied. Before proceeding with the pruning, it is helpful for us to take a careful look at the tree in Figure 4.3. Observe that many nodes are the offspring of the two nodes corresponding to complexity parameters α_4 and α_6. Considering the tree complexity, it is hard to imagine that we would keep these offspring in the final tree by any means. Thus, it makes sense here to perform a rough pruning first by cutting these offspring nodes before the formal pruning. Note, however, that α_1 through α_5 are smaller than α_6. Then, we ought to prune the offspring of all nodes corresponding to the complexity parameters α_1 through α_5. As a result, we have a subtree as presented in Figure 4.5, and all internal nodes in this tree are labeled. The new pruning procedure is applied to this smaller tree instead. Obviously, this step is not needed for an automated computer program.

As described above, we need to assign a statistic to each internal node. We accomplish it with two steps. First, we assign a raw statistic to each internal node. For example, we have the following 2×2 table for the root node:

	Term	Preterm	
Left Node	640	70	710
Right Node	3016	135	3151
	3656	205	3861

From this table, we calculated a relative risk (RR) of preterm as
$$(70/710)/(135/3151) = 2.3.$$

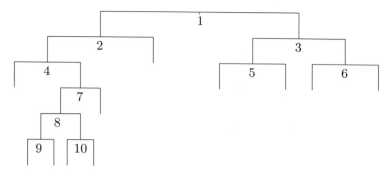

FIGURE 4.5. A roughly pruned subtree from Figure 4.3

Then, the logarithm of the relative risk is 0.833. Note also that the standard error for the log relative risk is approximately

$$\sqrt{1/70 - 1/710 + 1/135 - 1/3151} = 0.141.$$

See Agresti (1990, p. 56). Hence, the Studentized log relative risk is

$$0.833/0.141 = 5.91.$$

This Studentized log relative risk will be used as the raw statistic for the root node. Likewise, we can calculate the raw statistics for all internal nodes as reported in Table 4.4.

Next, for each internal node we replace the raw statistic with the maximum of the raw statistics over its offspring internal nodes if the latter is greater. For instance, the raw value 1.52 is replaced with 1.94 for node 4; here, 1.94 is the maximum of 1.47, 1.35, 1.94, 1.60, corresponding to nodes 7, 8, 9, and 10. The reassigned maximum node statistic is displayed in the third row of Table 4.4. We see that the maximum statistic has seven distinct values: 1.60, 1.69, 1.94, 2.29, 3.64, 3.72, and 5.91, each of which results in a subtree. Thus, we have a sequence of eight (7+1) nested subtrees, including the original tree in Figure 4.5. The seven subtrees are presented in Figure 4.6.

Figure 4.7 plots the sizes of the eight subtrees against their node statistics. If we use 1.96 as the threshold (corresponding to a significance level

TABLE 4.4. Statistics for Internal Nodes

Node #	1	2	3	4	5
Raw Statistic	5.91	2.29	3.72	1.52	3.64
Max. Statistic	5.91	2.29	3.72	1.94	3.64
Node #	6	7	8	9	10
Raw Statistic	1.69	1.47	1.35	1.94	1.60
Max. Statistic	1.69	1.94	1.94	1.94	1.60

46   4. Classification Trees for a Binary Response

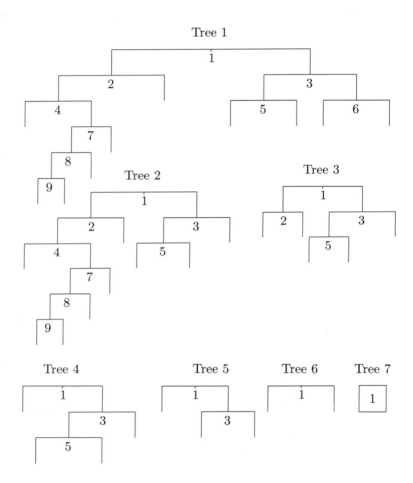

FIGURE 4.6. A sequence of nested subtrees

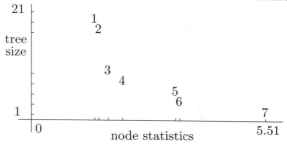

FIGURE 4.7. Tree size versus internal node statistics

of 0.05), tree 3 would be chosen as the final tree. Also, Figure 4.7 seems to suggest a kink at tree 3 or 4. Interestingly, tree 4 was selected by the pruning procedure introduced in Section 4.2.3 when $c(0|1) = 18$. See the discussion in the end of Section 4.4. Therefore, the alternative approach described here may be used as a guide to the cost selection of $c(0|1)$.

En route to determining the final tree structure, we must remember that interpretations are paramountly important. Note that the tree selection is based on a resubstitution estimate of relative risk. This estimate is potentially biased upward, because the splits are chosen by the impurity function, and the impurity relates closely to the relative risk. As a consequence of the selection bias, we cannot rely on the resubstitution estimate to interpret the tree results. In Section 4.6 we describe a way to adjust for the bias based on Zhang et al. (1996).

4.6 Localized Cross-Validation

As mentioned earlier, a selected split results in the following 2×2 table:

	Preterm	
	yes	no
Left Node	a	b
Right Node	c	d

$a/(a+b) \Big/ c/(c+d) > 1$

Without loss of generality, assume that $a(c+d)/(c(a+b)) > 1$. That is, the left node has higher risk than the right node. Let the true mean frequency counts be a^*, b^*, c^*, and d^* when we apply the selected split to an independent, identically distributed sample with the same number of term and preterm subjects, namely, $a+c = a^*+c^*$ and $b+d = b^*+d^*$. The selection bias implies that $I\!\!E(a) > a^*$ and $I\!\!E(d) > d^*$. In words, a and d are on average greater than a^* and d^*, respectively. We use a cross-validation procedure to estimate the degrees of overshoot in a and d. We view it as a localized procedure, because the cross-validation is performed among the subjects within the node of interest.

→ estimated agreement

A key idea is that the bias is a result of the selection process, and it is not specific to the cutoff value of the selected split. Suppose that we divide the sample in a node into learning and test subsamples. Using the learning sample, we can find a split that maximizes the impurity and leads to a 2×2 table T_l. Then, we apply the selected split to the test sample and derive another 2×2 table T_t. We can use the differences in the frequency counts between T_l and T_t to estimate the bias, $a - a^*$ and $d - d^*$.

Formally, we randomly divide the population of interest into v subpopulations. For instance, if $v = 5$, let $\mathcal{L}_i$ ($i = 1, 2, 3, 4, 5$) denote each of the 5 subpopulations and $\mathcal{L}_{(-i)}$ ($i = 1, 2, 3, 4, 5$) the sample after removing $\mathcal{L}_i$. We use $\mathcal{L}_{(-1)}$ to select a split s_1^* over the originally selected covariate; s_1^* results in two 2×2 tables, T_1 and $T_{(-1)}$:

	$T_{(-1)}$ Preterm			T_1 Preterm	
	yes	no		yes	no
Left Node	$a_{(-1)}$	$b_{(-1)}$	Left Node	a_1	b_1
Right Node	$c_{(-1)}$	$d_{(-1)}$	Right Node	c_1	d_1

We can always redefine the nodes for $T_{(-1)}$ in such a way that

$$\frac{a_{(-1)}(c_{(-1)} + d_{(-1)})}{c_{(-1)}(a_{(-1)} + b_{(-1)})} > 1,$$

and adjust T_1 accordingly. Next, we repeat this same process for all i and estimate the bias in a by the maximum of $\frac{1}{4}\sum_1^5 a_{(-i)} - \sum_1^5 a_i$ and $a - 0.5$ to guarantee that the frequency is positive. Similarly, we estimate the bias in d by the maximum of $\frac{1}{4}\sum_1^5 d_{(-i)} - \sum_1^5 d_i$ and $d - 0.5$. We correct the frequency counts by subtracting the corresponding bias and computing the relative risk and its standard error using these values.

For example, the adjusted 2×2 table for the root node in Figure 4.5 is

	Term	Preterm	
Left Node	682	70	752
Right Node	2973	135	3108
	3656	205	3861

Then, the cross-validation estimate of relative risk is

$$(70/752)/(135/3108) = 2.14,$$

which is a little smaller than the resubstitution estimate of 2.3. Meanwhile, the standard error of the log cross-validation estimate is approximately

$$\sqrt{1/70 - 1/752 + 1/135 - 1/3108} = 0.1414.$$

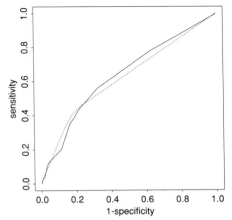

FIGURE 4.8. Comparison of ROC curves obtained by the tree structure and logistic regression model

Hence, the approximate 95% confidence interval for the relative risk is

$$(2.14\exp(-1.96*0.1414), 2.14\exp(1.96*0.1414)) = (1.62, 2.82).$$

Similarly, we can calculate the cross-validation estimate of relative risk for each internal node as shown in Figure 2.4.

4.7 Comparison Between Tree-Based and Logistic Regression Analyses

To compare the predictive power of the tree structure with the logistic regression model established in (3.3), we draw two ROC curves in Figure 4.8. The area under the curve is 0.622 for the tree-based model and 0.637 for the logistic model. When these models are applied to future test samples, their predictive power is expected to be even lower. Therefore, it is obvious from these ROC curves that there is much that needs to be done to improve our understanding of the determinants of preterm deliveries. For example, new risk factors should be sought.

Here, we describe two analytic strategies that are worth considering in tree-based analyses. Recall that we used only one predictor at a time when partitioning a node. In principle, a linear combination of the predictors can also be considered to split a node. The shortcomings with such an extension are threefold: (a) It is computationally difficult to find an optimal combination at the time of splitting. Partial solutions have been proposed in the literature. (b) The resulting split is not as intuitive as before. This is practically problematic. A Boolean summary of routes to a given terminal

TABLE 4.5. Definition of Dummy Variables from Terminal Nodes in Figure 2.4

Variable label	Specification
z_{13}	Black, unemployed
z_{14}	Black, employed
z_{15}	non-Black, ≤ 4 pregnancies, DES not used
z_{16}	non-Black, ≤ 4 pregnancies, DES used
z_{17}	non-Black, > 4 pregnancies

node assignment is closer to narrative disclosure and graspable by the end user. Linear combinations—unless they define a new scale—are not readily interpretable. (c) The combination is much more likely to be missing than its individual components. Thus, the optimality of the selected combination is dubious. Given these drawbacks, an exhaustive search for an optimal linear combination may not be worthwhile.

To make a more efficient use of data, to seek a more accurate predictive rule, and in the meantime, to avoid unjustifiable computational complications, it is a good idea to combine the logistic regression models and the tree-based models. The first approach is to take the linear equation derived from the logistic regression as a new predictor. Not surprisingly, this new predictor is generally more powerful than any individual predictor. In the present application, the new predictor is defined as

$$x_{16} = -2.344 - 0.076x_6 + 0.699z_6 + 0.115x_{11} + 1.539z_{10}. \qquad (4.13)$$

See Table 2.1 and equation (3.3) for the variable specification and the predicted risk equation. Figure 4.9 displays the final tree, which makes use of both the original and the created predictors. It is interesting to note a few points from Figure 4.9: (a) Education shows a protective effect, particularly for those with college or higher education. Not only does education participate in the derivation of x_{16} defined in (4.13), but itself also appears on the left-hand side of Figure 4.9. It did not appear, however, in Figure 2.4. (b) Age has merged as a risk factor. In the fertility literature, whether a women is at least 35 years old is a common standard for pregnancy screening. The threshold of 32 in Figure 4.9 is close to this common-sense choice. (c) The risk of delivering preterm babies is not monotonic with respect to the combined score x_{16}. In particular, the risk is lower when $-2.837 < x_{16} \leq -2.299$ than when $-2.299 < x_{16} \leq -2.062$. To the contrary, monotonicity holds when the risk is predicted with the logistic equation (3.3). The ROC curve for the new classification tree is shown in Figure 4.10, and the area under this curve is 0.661. We achieved some, but not much, improvement in predictive power. The second approach is to run the logistic regression after a tree is grown. For example, based on the tree displayed in Figure 2.4, we can create five dummy variables, each of which corresponds to one of the five terminal

4.7 Comparison Between Tree-Based and Logistic Regression Analyses 51

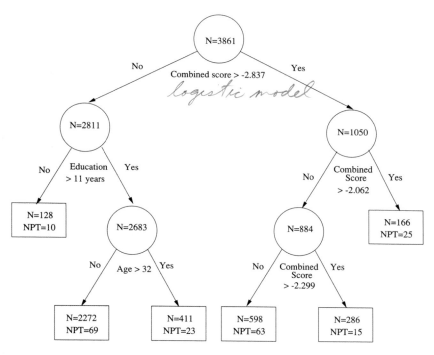

FIGURE 4.9. The final tree structure making use of the equation from the logistic regression. N: sample size; NPT: number of preterm cases.

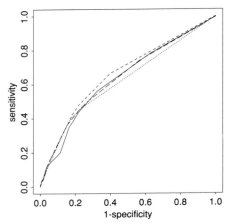

FIGURE 4.10. Comparison of ROC curves obtained by the tree structure (dotted), logistic regression model (solid), and their hybrid (the first approach, shortly-dashed; the second approach, long-dashed)

nodes. Table 4.5 specifies these five dummy variables. In particular, the leftmost terminal node contains 512 unemployed Black women. The dummy variable, z_{13}, equals 1 for the 512 unemployed Black women and 0 for the rest. Next, we include these five dummy variables, z_{13} to z_{17}, in addition to the fifteen predictors, x_1 to x_{15}, in Table 2.1 and rebuild a logistic regression model. The new equation for the predicted risk is

$$\hat{\theta} = \frac{\exp(-1.341 - 0.071x_6 - 0.885z_{15} + 1.016z_{16})}{1 + \exp(-1.341 - 0.071x_6 - 0.885z_{15} + 1.016z_{16})}. \quad (4.14)$$

Looking at it carefully, we see that the equation above is very similar to equation (3.3). The variables z_{15} and z_{16} are an interactive version of z_6, x_{11}, and z_{10}. The coefficient for x_6 is nearly intact. If any, the difference lies in the use of an additive or an interactive model. As expected, the ROC curve corresponding to (4.14) is very close to that from (3.3) as displayed in Figure 4.10. The area under the new curve is 0.642, which is narrowly higher than 0.639.

It is important to realize that our comparison of predictive power is based on ROC curves that were derived by the resubstitution approach. The same precision usually does not hold when the prediction rule is applied to a test sample. Although we demonstrated some potential improvement of precision by the hybrids of the tree-based and logistic regression models, the same degree of improvement is possible, but not guaranteed, for a test sample.

4.8 Missing Data

We have described major issues involved in the tree-growing and pruning steps, assuming no missing data. In many applications, however, missing data occur. We introduce two notable approaches to dealing with missing data. One approach makes use of surrogate splits (Breiman et al., 1984, Section 5.3). Zhang et al. (1996) named the other the "missings together" (MT) approach, which was also implemented by Clark and Pregibon (1992). Depending on the purpose of data analysis, data analysts may choose either approach. Since the MT approach is relatively straightforward, we describe it first.

4.8.1 Missings Together Approach

The key idea of the MT approach is this. Suppose that we attempt to split node τ by variable x_j and that x_j is missing for a number of subjects. The MT approach forces all of these subjects to the same daughter node of node τ. In contrast, both daughter nodes may contain some of these subjects by using surrogate splits instead.

Consider variable x_j. If it is a nominal variable with k levels, the missing value is regarded as an additional level. Then, x_j has $k+1$ levels. On the other hand, when x_j has a natural order, we first make two copies $x_j^{(1)}$ and $x_j^{(2)}$ of x_j. Suppose that $x_j = (x_{j1}, \ldots, x_{jN})'$. If the component x_{ji} is missing, set $x_{ji}^{(1)} = -\infty$ and $x_{ji}^{(2)} = \infty$. Here, $-\infty$ and ∞ can be any numbers that are, respectively, smaller and larger than observable x_j.

For example, let us take $x_j = (2, -4, \text{NA}, 1, 7, \text{NA})'$; here NA stands for missing values. Then,

$$x_j^{(1)} = (2, -4, -\infty, 1, 7, -\infty)' \text{ and } x_j^{(2)} = (2, -4, \infty, 1, 7, \infty)'.$$

Originally, x_j contributes three allowable splits, namely, (1) $x_j > -4$ versus $x_j \leq -4$; (2) $x_j > 1$ versus $x_j \leq 1$; and (3) $x_j > 2$ versus $x_j \leq 2$. If we want to put all subjects with missing x_j in the same node, we have the following seven allowable splits: (1) $x_j > -4$ or NA versus $x_j \leq -4$; (2) $x_j > 1$ or NA versus $x_j \leq 1$; (3) $x_j > 2$ or NA versus $x_j \leq 2$; (4) NA versus non-NA; (5) $x_j > -4$ versus $x_j \leq -4$ or NA; (6) $x_j > 1$ versus $x_j \leq 1$ or NA; (7) $x_j > 2$ versus $x_j \leq 2$ or NA. It is important to note that when $x_j^{(1)}$ is used as a splitting variable, it generates the first four allowable splits; and likewise, $x_j^{(2)}$ produces the last four allowable splits. Since both $x_j^{(1)}$ and $x_j^{(2)}$ can yield the fourth allowable split, they together result in the seven allowable splits as listed above. Because of this observation, we can replace x_j with its two variants $x_j^{(1)}$ and $x_j^{(2)}$ so that the subjects with missing x_j are sent to the same node.

Here are some of the advantages of the MT approach. It is very simple to implement. In fact, if we have a core recursive partition algorithm that assumes no missing data, we can still use the same algorithm without modification when the raw data contain missing values. The trick is that we can use the MT approach to prepare another data set with "complete" information. Lastly, we can easily trace where the subjects with missing information are located in a tree structure.

4.8.2 Surrogate Splits

Contributed by Breiman et al. (1984), surrogate splits is an important technique for handling missing data in tree-based methods. Let us imagine that race is missing for, say, 10 subjects in Figure 2.4. Since race is the splitting variable for the root node, we have a problem in deciding to which daughter node we send these 10 subjects. The "missings together" approach described above sends all 10 subjects to one daughter node. On the other hand, surrogate splits attempts to utilize the information in other predictors to assist us in making such a decision. For example, an obvious choice of replacing race is the second-best splitting variable, a so-called competitive split. The problem is that a competitive split does not necessarily offer a good replacement for race when race is missing. Therefore, it is a good idea to look for a predictor that is most similar to race in classifying the subjects. What, then, do we mean by "similar"? One measure of similarity between two splits suggested by Breiman et al. (1984) is the coincidence probability that the two splits send a subject to the same node. For instance, the 2 × 2 table below compares the split of "is age > 35?" with the selected race split.

	Black	Others
Age ≤ 35	702	8
Age > 35	3017	134

702+134=836 of 3,861 subjects are sent to the same node, and hence $836/3861 = 0.217$ can be used as an estimate for the coincidence probability of these two splits. In general, prior information should be incorporated in estimating the coincidence probability when the subjects are not randomly drawn from a general population, such as in case-control studies. In such cases, we estimate the coincidence probability with

$$I\!P\{Y=0\}M_0(\tau)/N_0(\tau) + I\!P\{Y=1\}M_1(\tau)/N_1(\tau),$$

where $N_j(\tau)$ is the total number of class j subjects in node τ and $M_j(\tau)$ is the number of class j subjects in node τ that are sent to the same daughters by the two splits; here $j=0$ (normal) and 1(abnormal). $I\!P\{Y=0\}$ and $I\!P\{Y=1\}$ are the priors to be specified. Usually, $I\!P\{Y=1\}$ is the prevalence rate of a disease under investigation and $I\!P\{Y=0\} = 1 - I\!P\{Y=1\}$.

Definition 4.1 *The Best Surrogate Split*

For any split s^*, split s' is the best surrogate split of s^* when s' yields the greatest coincidence probability with s^* over all allowable splits based on different predictors.

It is not unlikely, though, that the predictor that yields the best surrogate split may also be missing. Then, we have to look for the second best, and so on. If our purpose is to build an automatic classification rule (e.g., Goldman et al., 1982, 1996), it is not difficult for a computer to keep track of the list of surrogate splits. However, the same task may not be easy for humans. Surrogate splits could contain useful information for the analyst who is trying to extract maximal insight from the data in the course of determining the final tree. On the other hand, due to the limited space, surrogate splits are rarely published in the literature, and hence their usefulness is hampered by this practical limitation.

There is no guarantee that surrogate splits improve the predictive power of a particular split as compared to a random split. In such cases, the surrogate splits should be discarded.

If surrogate splits are used, the user should take full advantage of them. In particular, a thorough examination of the best surrogate splits may reveal other important predictors that are absent from the final tree structure, and it may also provide alternative tree structures that in principle can have a lower misclassification cost than the final tree, because the final tree is selected in a stepwise manner and is not necessarily a local optimizer in any sense.

4.9 Tree Stability

One of the most serious concerns in applying the tree-based methods is tree stability. For example, if we take a random sample of 3,861 with replacement from the Yale Pregnancy Outcome Study, what is the chance that we come to the same tree as presented Figure 2.4? Unfortunately, this chance is not so great. To be fair, however, we should acknowledge that this is not an uncommon phenomenon. All stepwise model selections potentially suffer from the same problem. Although model stability is a generally important issue and deserves serious attention, it would be ironic for us to question the tree stability while not being concerned with the model instability in general. For example, we do not see many papers that employ stepwise logistic regression explore alternative model structures.

Despite the general model instability, the tree structure is not as shaky as it looks. In practice, the real cause of concern regarding tree stability is the psychological effect of the appearance of a tree. Based on the evidence presented by Breiman et al. (1984, Section 5.5.2), competitive trees of different appearances can give fairly stable and consistent final predictions.

56   4. Classification Trees for a Binary Response

So, tree stability is a reasonable concern and should be examined in the same way as in the use of other model selection procedures, but it should not discourage us from using the tree-based methods.

When using a tree-based method, we usually either have a test sample or apply cross-validation. We can investigate tree stability by studying the tree from the test sample or the trees generated during cross-validation. Certain parts of tree are more stable than others, and hence it is a useful practice to distinguish the less stable parts from the stable ones; see, e.g., Zhang et al. (1996). The justification of the less stable part may require more data.

Thanks to computer technology, it becomes feasible now for us to examine a massive number of alternative trees. Bayesian approaches aided by Markov Chain Monte Carlo (MCMC) have emerged recently; see, e.g., Chipman et al. (1998) and Denison et al. (1998). The idea is to obtain a posterior likelihood for a large number of trees and select a tree with the highest likelihood using the MCMC algorithm. The difficulty is, however, that many priors must be specified, and this could make it impractical to popularize the use of Bayesian CART. Nevertheless, Bayesian ideas are fruitful, particularly if the selection and justification of the priors could be substantially simplified and standardized. In addition, Bayesian methodology could open new possibilities to explore a forest of trees within which all trees have a reasonable high credential in terms of the posterior probability. The size and the quality of the forest can provide information with regard to the tree stability.

4.10 Implementation*

We have seen that a large number of splits must be searched in order to grow a tree. Here, we address the computational issue of designing a fast search algorithm.

Recall that the partitioning process is the same for all internal nodes including the root node. Therefore, it suffices to explain the process with the root node. Moreover, we encounter really two types of predictors: ordered and unordered. For simplicity, we use daily alcohol intake in Table 2.1 as an example for ordered predictors. This variable, x_{13}, takes a value from 0, 1, 2, and 3. The race variable, x_3, in the same table will serve as an example of nominal (not ordered) predictors.

For each of x_3 and x_{13} we need to construct a matrix that holds the numbers of normal and abnormal subjects at every level of the predictor. The two corresponding matrices are:

4.10 Implementation*

Matrix A_3(root) for x_3

		Whites	Blacks	Hispanics	Asians	Others
y	0	2880	640	103	20	13
	1	128	70	6	1	0

Matrix A_{13}(root) for x_{13}

		0	1	2	3
y	0	1113	1	2245	297
	1	76	0	110	19

As displayed in Table 2.2, x_3 generates $2^{5-1} - 1 = 15$ allowable splits; here the number "5" in the exponent is the number of the levels of x_3. The question is, How can we search over these fifteen choices efficiently? To this end, we introduce a binary array of length 5 as follows,

Level:	Whites	Blacks	Hispanics	Asians	Others
Array:	1	0	1	0	1

where a bit "1" indicates that a subject who has the corresponding race group goes to the left daughter node. Hence, the array above implies that 3,008 Whites, 109 Hispanics, and 13 others are in the left node, while the remaining 731 Blacks and Asians are in the right node.

Each of the fifteen allowable splits corresponds to a distinct assignment of bits for the array. In fact, we know that any integer from 1 to 15 can be expressed in a binary format as displayed in Table 4.6. If we take 7 from Table 4.6, its binary representation is 00111. This array indicates that 3,008 whites and 710 blacks should be in the right daughter node. The use of the binary representation following the original order of 1 to 15 is a little troublesome, however, for the following reason.

Note that the binary representation for 1 is 00001. Thus, the first allowable split is to put the 13 subjects in the "others" racial group in the left node and the remaining 3,848 subjects in the right node. Now, the binary representation of 2 is 00010. Then, the next split would exchange node assignments for the 13 others and the 21 Asians. Thus, from the first to the second splits, two groups of subjects are involved. As a matter of fact, three groups of subjects must be switched as we move from the third to the fourth split, because the binary representations of 3 and 4 differ by three bits. The housekeeping for these movements is not convenient. Fortunately, there is a simple algorithm that can rearrange the order of the integers such that the binary representation changes only one bit as we go from one integer to the next. This rearrangement is also given in Table 4.6. The importance of the rearrangement is that only one group needs to be reallocated as we evaluate the splits from one to the next. This makes it very simple to update the changes, and in fact, it cannot be simpler.

58   4. Classification Trees for a Binary Response

TABLE 4.6. Binary Representation of Integers

Original order		Rearranged order	
Integer	Binary	Integer	Binary
1	00001	1	00001
2	00010	3	00011
3	00011	2	00010
4	00100	6	00110
5	00101	7	00111
6	00110	5	00101
7	00111	4	00100
8	01000	12	01100
9	01001	13	01101
10	01010	15	01111
11	01011	14	01110
12	01100	10	01010
13	01101	11	01011
14	01110	9	01001
15	01111	8	01000

Since the first binary array under the rearranged order is 00001, the first split is still the one that sends the 13 others to the left node and the remaining 3,848 subjects to the right. Then, matrix A_3(root) breaks into two parts:

		Left	Right			
		Others	Whites	Blacks	Hispanics	Asians
y	0	13	2880	640	103	20
	1	0	128	70	6	1

The impurities for the left and right daughter nodes are respectively 0 and 0.208. Thus, the goodness of the split is

$$0.2075 - \frac{3848}{3861} * 0.208 - \frac{13}{3861} * 0 = 0.0002,$$

where 0.2075 is the impurity of the root node.

The second binary array under the rearranged order is 00011. Hence, the 21 Asian subjects join the left node in the second split. The record is then modified to:

		Left		Right		
		Asians	Others	Whites	Blacks	Hispanics
y	0	20	13	2880	640	103
	1	1	0	128	70	6

The goodness of this split is 0.00006. Analogously, we can evaluate the goodness of the remaining thirteen splits. In general, when the matrix "A" is prepared for the node to be split, it is very fast to find the best candidate split for a particular nominal predictor, because the number of computing steps is proportional to the number of allowable splits, which is rarely above 127, corresponding to a nominal predictor with 8 levels. Since it is unusual to use recursive partitioning with many fewer than 127 subjects, the number of computing steps will not be beyond the magnitude of the sample size. Importantly, we need to create the matrix only for the root node, because the corresponding matrices for the subsequent nodes can be obtained as a by-product of the search for the best split.

A similar process applies to finding the best candidate split from x_{13} or any other ordered predictors. First, we send all subjects for which $x_{13} = 0$ to the left daughter node, because 0 is the minimum of the observed x_{13}. Hence, $A_{13}(\text{root})$ is divided into:

		Left		Right	
		0	1	2	3
y	0	1113	1	2245	297
	1	76	0	110	19

This split gives rise to a goodness of split of 0.0005. Next, the subjects whose x_{13} equals 1 move to the left node, because 1 is adjacent to 0. Then, the subjects with $x_{13} = 2$ are switched to the left node, and so on. Therefore, whenever we proceed to the next split, one more slice (i.e., column) of $A_{13}(\text{root})$ is moved to the left node. The number of moves depends on the number of the distinctly observed data points for the predictor; in the worst case, it is in the order of the sample size. Therefore, after $A_{13}(\text{root})$ is determined, the number of needed computing steps is at most a constant proportion of the sample size. The constant is smaller than 10. Moreover, when we split the subsequent nodes, the number of subjects becomes smaller and smaller. In fact, for a given predictor the total number of computing steps for splitting all nodes in the same layer is usually smaller than that for splitting the root node.

To conclude, the total number of computing steps needed to construct a tree of d layers is about $cpn\log(n) + 10dpn$, where p is the number of predictors, n is the sample size, and the term, $cpn\log(n)$, results from preparing the A matrices. Obviously, the second term generally dominates the first term.

5
Risk-Factor Analysis Using Tree-Based Stratification

In epidemiologic studies, one of the most frequently encountered issues is to evaluate the association between a set of putative risk factors and a disease outcome, controlling for another set of potential confounders. In this chapter, we illustrate how to apply the tree-based method in this regard. The discussion is mostly adopted from Zhang and Bracken (1996).

5.1 Background

Spontaneous abortion, one of the most difficult reproductive outcomes to study using epidemiologic methods, will be the outcome of interest; see, e.g., Zhang and Bracken (1996). The difficulties in this area of research include failure to detect a large proportion (perhaps majority) of spontaneous abortions and the large number of known and suspected confounding risk factors that must be considered before evaluating the possible role of new factors. The situation is shared by many diseases such as cancer, AIDS, and coronary heart disease.

Our illustrative data come from a continuation project of the Yale Pregnancy Outcome Study. The study population consists of women receiving prenatal care at 11 private obstetrical practices and two health maintenance organizations in Southern Connecticut during the period 1988 to 1991. They were 2,849 women who had initial home interviews during 5 to 16 weeks of pregnancy between April 5, 1988 and December 1, 1991, and whose pregnancies resulted in a singleton live birth or spontaneous

TABLE 5.1. List of Putative Risk Factors

Characteristics	No. of subjects	%‡
Currently employed		
No	638	5.3
Yes	2211	4.6
Standing 2+ hours at work daily		
No	2559	4.6
Yes	290	5.9
Walking 2+ hours at work daily		
No	1894	4.9
Yes	955	4.5
Sitting 2+ hours at work daily		
No	1230	5.2
Yes	1619	4.4
Vibration at work		
No	2756	4.7
Yes	93	5.4
Commute to work		
No	705	4.8
Yes	2144	4.7
Reaching over the shoulders on the job		
No	1584	4.5
<1/day	530	4.5
1+/day	735	5.4
Carrying loads over 20 lbs on the job		
No	2154	4.4
<1/day	318	3.8
1+/day	386	7.3

‡ Percentage of spontaneous abortions

abortion. Initial home interviews were conducted early in the pregnancy so that evaluation of spontaneous abortion in mid-to-late first and second trimesters would be possible. A more detailed description of the study design has appeared elsewhere (Bracken et al. 1995).

Of particular interest are the effects of the eight job-related putative risk factors as listed in Table 5.1 on spontaneous abortions. Also presented in this table is the information regarding the characteristics of the study subgroups defined by the individual risk factor. To evaluate these risk factors, Zhang and Bracken included eighteen potential confounders that might alter the association of interest. As given in Table 5.2, these potential confounders have been examined frequently in the relevant literature; see Zhang and Bracken (1996) for more information. The list of confounders concentrates on maternal characteristics before pregnancy. It includes de-

TABLE 5.2. Potential Confounding Factors

Variable name	Label	Type	Range/levels
Maternal age	x_1	Continuous	13–45
Years of education	x_2	Continuous	8–20
Marital status	x_3	Nominal	Married, Cohabiting Separated/Widowed Divorced, Not married
Race	x_4	Nominal	White, Black Hispanic, Asian Others
Mother's height	x_5	Continuous	51–73 (inches)
Years of smoking	x_6	Continuous	0–25
Smoked marijuana	x_7	Binary	Yes, No
Exposure to someone else's marijuana use	x_8	Binary	Yes, No
Used cocaine	x_9	Binary	Yes, No
Used birth control	x_{10}	Binary	Yes, No
Smoked	x_{11}	Binary	Yes, No
Stopped smoking	x_{12}	Binary	Yes, No
Gravidity	x_{13}	Ordinal	0–2, 3+
Infertility	x_{14}	Binary	Yes, No
Induced abortion	x_{15}	Binary	Yes, No
Stillbirth	x_{16}	Binary	Yes, No
Spontaneous abortion	x_{17}	Binary	Yes, No
Ectopic spontaneous abortion	x_{18}	Binary	Yes, No

mographic and behavioral factors as well as ones related to pregnancy history.

5.2 The Analysis

The analysis proceeds in four steps. The first step evaluates the marginal association between spontaneous abortion and each of the eight risk factors. In the second step, the tree-based method is applied, using the 18 confounders in Table 5.2 as predictors. As a result, the study sample is stratified into seven subgroups. Then, Mantel–Haenszel's method is employed in the stratified samples to derive adjusted relative risks. Logistic regression is conducted for the purpose of comparison.

First, we examine the marginal association between spontaneous abortion and the eight putative risk factors using the χ^2 test. Table 5.3 features the crude relative risks (RR) and their 95% confidence intervals (CI). "Car-

64   5. Risk-Factor Analysis Using Tree-Based Stratification

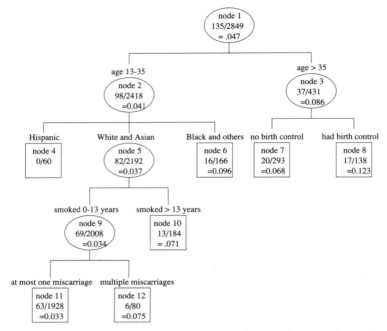

FIGURE 5.1. The tree structure for the sample stratification. Reproduced from Figure 1 of Zhang and Bracken (1996).

rying loads over 20 lbs on the job" shows significant marginal association at the level of 0.05. This factor has 3 categories: (a) those who did not carry loads over 20 lbs daily at work (unemployed women included); (b) those who carried loads over 20 lbs less than once per day; and (c) those who carried loads over 20 lbs at least once a day. Seventy-five, 11, and 14 percent of the subjects, respectively, fall in each of these categories. Although there is hardly any difference in the rates of spontaneous abortion between the first two categories, the difference is significant between the first two and the third. Using the group not carrying loads over 20 lbs as the reference, the relative risk due to carrying loads over 20 lbs at least once daily is 1.71, and its 95% confidence interval is (1.25, 2.32).

As the second step, we make use of the tree-based method to stratify the study sample into a number of meaningful and homogeneous subgroups, each of which corresponds to a terminal node in the tree structure. In this exercise, we use the alternative pruning approach described in Section 4.5 and adopt the missings together strategy of Section 4.8 to handle the missing data. Similar to the tree constructed in Figure 2.4, we end up with the tree in Figure 5.1 for the present data.

Figure 5.1 can be read as follows. Node 1 is the entire study population of 2,849 pregnant women. The overall rate of spontaneous abortion is 4.7%. This sample is first divided into two age groups: 13–35 and >35.

TABLE 5.3. Marginal Associations Between Spontaneous Abortion and the Putative Risk Factors

Factor	No. of subjects	%[‡]	RR	CI
Currently employed				
No	638	5.3	Reference	
Yes	2211	4.6	0.86	0.59–1.25
Standing 2+ hours at work daily				
No	2559	4.6	Reference	
Yes	290	5.9	1.27	0.78–2.08
Walking 2+ hours at work daily				
No	1894	4.9	Reference	
Yes	955	4.5	0.93	0.65–1.32
Sitting 2+ hours at work daily				
No	1230	5.2	Reference	
Yes	1619	4.4	0.84	0.61–1.17
Vibration at work				
No	2756	4.7	Reference	
Yes	93	5.4	1.14	0.48–2.72
Commute to work				
No	705	4.8	Reference	
Yes	2144	4.7	0.98	0.67–1.43
Reaching over the shoulders on the job				
No	1584	4.5	Reference	
<1/day	530	4.5	1.01	0.64–1.59
1+/day	735	5.4	1.21	0.83–1.77
Carrying loads over 20 lbs on the job				
No	2154	4.4	Reference	
<1/day	318	3.8	0.85	0.47–1.54
1+/day	386	7.3	(1.64)	1.09–2.46

[‡] Percentage of spontaneous abortions
Based on Table 2 of Zhang and Bracken (1996)

The younger group is called node 2 and the older group node 3. Note that the rates of spontaneous abortion in nodes 2 and 3 become 4.1% and 8.6%, respectively. Age 35 is a traditional choice of age grouping for perinatal studies, and it is an interesting coincidence that the computer also found the traditional choice to be optimal. Then, we continue to split nodes 2 and 3. The greatest reduction of impurity is found through race for the younger group as node 2 is divided into three ethnic groups. Usually, the tree-based method splits a node into two subgroups only. The computer selected the racial split as: "White, Asian, and Hispanic" versus "Black and others." Since there was no spontaneous abortion reported among the 60 Hispanic pregnant women, we separated them from White and Asian women. The older group (node 3) is split by the prior use of any birth control.

Only one node, number 5 in the third level of the tree, is further divided. It is the group of young, White or Asian women, constituting the majority of the study sample. Their risk of spontaneous abortion is 3.7%. For them, the partition is whether they have smoked more than 13 years. Finally, if they have smoked for less than 13 years, they would be in node 9, which is again divided into nodes 11 and 12 according to previous history of spontaneous abortion (≤ 1 versus ≥ 2).

As identified by rectangles, there are seven terminal nodes (numbers 4, 6, 7, 8, 10, 11, and 12) in Figure 5.1. Since every study subject eventually falls into one terminal node (for example, a woman older than 35 belongs to terminal node 7 if she did not take any birth control), the seven terminal nodes define seven strata of the entire study sample.

Next, we use Mantel–Haenszel's method (Mantel and Haenszel, 1959) to find the adjusted relative risks based on the stratification defined by Figure 5.1. To explain this process, we use employment as an example. For each terminal node, we have a 2×2 table in which the columns correspond to the outcome (yes, no) and the rows to the exposure (yes, no) as follows:

a_i	b_i	n_{1i}
c_i	d_i	n_{0i}
m_{1i}	m_{0i}	n_i

$i = 1, \ldots, 7$. As a result, we have the following seven 2×2 tables:

0	46		45	1461		18	204		9	127
0	14		18	404		2	69		4	44

4	45		13	123		12	104
2	29		3	27		5	17

With the analogy to the Mantel and Haenszel (1959) statistic, our summary relative risk estimate is

$$r = \frac{\sum_{i=1}^{7} a_i n_{0i}/n_i}{\sum_{i=1}^{7} c_i n_{1i}/n_i}.$$

5.2 The Analysis

Applying this formula to the seven tables, we have

$$r = \frac{0 + \frac{45*422}{1928} + \frac{18*71}{293} + \frac{9*48}{184} + \frac{4*31}{80} + \frac{13*30}{166} + \frac{12*22}{138}}{0 + \frac{18*1506}{1928} + \frac{2*222}{293} + \frac{4*136}{184} + \frac{2*49}{80} + \frac{3*136}{166} + \frac{5*116}{138}} = 0.85.$$

The limits of $100(1-\alpha)\%$ confidence interval for the relative risk can be obtained from $r^{(1 \pm z_{\alpha/2}/\chi)}$, where $z_{\alpha/2}$ is the upper $\alpha/2$ percentile of the standard normal distribution, and the χ^2-statistic, developed by Cochran (1954) and Mantel and Haenszel (1959), can be computed as follows:

$$\chi^2 = \frac{(|\sum_{i=1}^{7}(a_i - A_i)| - 0.5)^2}{\sum_{i=1}^{7} V_i}, \tag{5.1}$$

where

$$A_i = \frac{n_{1i} m_{1i}}{n_i} \text{ and } V_i = \frac{n_{1i} n_{0i} m_{1i} m_{0i}}{n_i^2 (n_i - 1)},$$

$i = 1, \ldots, 7$. For the present seven tables, $\chi^2 = 1.093$, giving a 95% confidence interval (0.62, 1.16) for the relative risk.

If the stratification were determined a priori without the help of the tree-based method, this approach of adjustment would be the same as the one used by Mills et al. (1991) and Giovannucci et al. (1995) among others. Moreover, if the linear discriminant analysis were used to stratify the data, it would be the approach proposed by Miettinen (1976). In all cases, the confounding factors are controlled through the strata. In other words, we use tree-based methods to reduce the data dimension of the confounding factors and to construct a filter for the evaluation of new risk factors. So, the first stage of analysis is the sample stratification based on the confounders, and the second stage is the calculation of the adjusted relative risk for the new risk factors.

As reported under the column of RR in Table 5.4, one risk factor showed significant effects. That is "carry load over 20 lbs at least once daily" [RR=1.71, 95% confidence interval= (1.25, 2.32)]. Nevertheless, a more modest risk factor is "reaching over the shoulders at least once daily" [RR=1.35, 95% confidence interval=(1.02, 1.78)]. Table 5.4 presents more detail on the association of the risk factors to spontaneous abortion. In this table, the adjusted RR is the Mantel–Haenszel estimate, and the adjusted odds ratio (OR) is from logistic regression.

For the purpose of comparison, Zhang and Bracken (1996) also reported analysis based on logistic regression. The model selection is not conventional. Instead, they made use of Figure 5.1. The main and the second-order interaction effects of the five variables (age, race, years of smoking, miscarriage, and use of birth control) that stratify the study sample are included in the initial logistic regression. A forward stepwise procedure selected a logistic model with three significant terms: age (p-value = 0.002), race (Whites and Asians, p-value = 0.04), and race (Hispanic, p-value =

TABLE 5.4. Adjusted Relative Risk and Odds Ratio of Spontaneous Abortion Attributed by Individual Putative Risk Factor

Factor	RR	CI	OR	CI
Currently employed				
No	Reference			
Yes	0.85	0.62–1.16	0.82	0.55–1.23
Standing 2+ hours at work daily				
No	Reference			
Yes	1.27	0.83–1.94	1.28	0.76–2.17
Walking 2+ hours at work daily				
No	Reference			
Yes	0.97	0.60–1.56	0.95	0.65–1.38
Sitting 2+ hours at work daily				
No	Reference			
Yes	.81	0.63–1.05	0.80	0.57–1.14
Vibration at work				
No	Reference			
Yes	1.11	0.58–2.13	1.11	0.44–2.80
Commuting to work				
No	Reference			
Yes	0.96	0.59–1.54	0.96	0.65–1.44
Reaching over the shoulders on the job				
No	Reference			
<1/day	0.98	0.58–1.67	1.02	0.63–1.64
1+/day	1.35	1.02–1.78	1.30	0.87–1.95
Carrying loads over 20 lbs on the job				
No	Reference			
<1/day	0.91	0.43–1.93	0.87	0.47–1.61
1+/day	1.71	1.25–2.32	1.75	1.13–2.71

Based on Table 2 of Zhang and Bracken (1996)

0.01). Then, they examined eight additional logit models by adding and then deleting one of the eight putative risk factors, one at a time, into the selected 3-term logit model. The results are reported in the last two columns of Table 5.4. It is apparent from Tables 5.3 and 5.4 that the three estimates of risk (crude RR, adjusted RR, and adjusted OR) give very close answers. Therefore, for the present analysis, the eighteen potential confounders are proven not to be confounders.

In summary, Zhang and Bracken (1996) found that risk of spontaneous abortion increases as women carry loads over 20 lbs at least once a day, or reach over the shoulders at least once a day, neither of which is recognized as a risk factor in the extant literature. Hence, these occupational exposures merit additional study.

6
Analysis of Censored Data: Examples

6.1 Introduction

Censored survival time is the outcome of numerous studies. We select a few examples from the medical literature to give a glimpse of the scope of studies involving censored survival time. Although survival time is usually the time to death, it can be broadly referred to as the time to the occurrence of an event of interest. For example, age of onset for breast cancer can be interpreted as a survival time.

Example 6.1 Ansell et al. (1993) performed a tree-based survival analysis on 127 consecutive women with stage IIIB to stage IV ovarian cancer. Between November 1982 and July 1988, those patients had undergone surgical procedures as treatment for advanced ovarian cancer. The survival status of the patients was monitored from the time of the surgery to January 30, 1992. Eighty-four patients had died during this period of time, and the remaining 43 were still alive at the final date of the study. Hence, the survival time of the 43 alive patients was censored. The study goal is to scrutinize demographic and tumor-related prognostic (clinical, radiological, and biochemical) factors that predict survival. Based on their analysis, Ansell et al. defined three groups of patients with significantly (at the level of 0.05) different survival functions.

Example 6.2 From 1974 to 1989, 1,578 patients were entered in three Radiation Therapy Oncology Group malignant glioma trials. Curran et al. (1993) used this sample to examine the associations of survival time to pretreatment patient status and tumor characteristics, and treatment-related indicators. The survival time was calculated from the date of the treatment to November 1991. The pretreatment factors include age, performance status, and tumor histopathology. Extent of surgery is one of the five treatment-related variables. Using the recursive partitioning technique, the authors identified six subgroups with distinct survival durations. The most important stratification is whether or not the patient was younger than 50 years of age.

Example 6.3 The determinants of life span are complex and include genetic factors. To explore the effect of three ($H - 2^b$, $H - 2^k$, and $H - 2^d$) haplotypes on the T-cell functions and ultimately on survival, Salazar et. al (1995) conducted an experimental study using 1,537 mice that were born between April 14 and July 28, 1987. The experiment ended on February 2, 1991. During the experiment period, the survival durations of 130 mice (in addition to those that were still alive at the end) were censored (not observed) because of accidental drowning of 5 and sacrifice of 125 for immunologic studies. The authors found that males lived longer than females except for $H - 2^d$ homozygotes, for which there was no sign of significant difference at the level of 0.05.

What do Examples 6.1–6.3 have in common? As in Examples 1.1–1.6, the observations from every subject include a number of predictors such as prognostic factors in Example 6.1 and genetic components in Example 6.3. What makes it more special here is the outcome of interest, which is a clearly defined, but sometimes unobservable, survival time. Depending on the nature of study, the survival time, denoted by T, may be calculated from the time of the treatment (e.g, surgery in Example 6.1) or the time of birth (e.g., Example 6.3) to the time of death (or broadly, the time when an event occurs). Due to practical constraints, we are not able to observe all subjects until after death. Thus, all studies have a clearly defined end. For example, the last day is February 2, 1991, in Example 6.3. Sometimes, the end of study may be the day when a prespecified number of study subjects have died. Those subjects that were alive at the end of the study have a censored survival time. In other words, their survival times were actually longer than what we could observe. There are also other circumstances in which we cannot observe the relevant survival time. For instance, 130 mice in Example 6.3 died from a cause other than the one of interest. They would have survived longer if they had not been killed by accidents or been sacrificed. In many human clinical trials, some subjects may be lost before the end of the study because of various health conditions or inconvenience (e.g., having moved out of the study area).

Figure 6.1 elucidates two typical study designs and three common types of censoring. In panel (a), all subjects enter into a study at the same time. When the study ends on a planned date, type I censoring occurs. If the

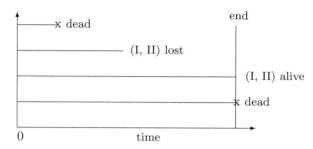
(a) All subjects enter into the study at the same time

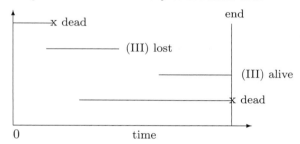
(b) Subjects enter into the study at the different times

FIGURE 6.1. Three types of censoring

study is terminated after a given number of subjects have died, we have type II censoring. For both types of censoring, subjects may be either alive at the end of study or lost to follow-up during the study period. In panel (b), subjects enter into a study at different times. The censoring is classified as type III. In almost all cases where the tree-based methods have been applied, types I and III, called random censoring, are involved. Type II censoring times among subjects are not independent. We will not discuss further the distinction between random and nonrandom censoring. All of these types are *right* censoring, or censoring to the right.

Although we do not pursue it here, left censoring and interval (double) censoring also arise in practice (e.g., Peto, 1973). Particularly in AIDS (acquired immunodeficiency syndrome) research, estimating the time from the HIV (human immunodeficiency virus) infection to the development of AIDS, called the incubation period, is very important to the control and prevention of AIDS (e.g., Brookmeyer, 1991). The difficulty is that the time of HIV infection is unknown and the incubation period is left-censored. Supposing that the duration from the onset of HIV infection to the AIDS death is of interest, interval censoring occurs.

In summary, we cannot observe the survival time for all study subjects. To take into account the fact of survival being censored, we use δ to indicate whether a subject's survival is observed (if it is one) or censored (if it is zero). Although the survival time is the sole outcome, it involves two response variables: the observed time, denoted by Y, and the censoring indicator. In the absence of censoring, the observed time is the survival time, and hence $Y = T$. Otherwise, the observed time is the censoring time, denoted by U. The relationship among T, Y, U, and δ is $Y = \min(T, U)$ and $\delta = I(Y = T)$, where $I(\cdot)$ is an indicator function defined as follows:

$$I(A) = \begin{cases} 1 & \text{if condition } A \text{ is met}, \\ 0 & \text{otherwise}. \end{cases} \quad (6.1)$$

We will explain later how to use the ideas expressed in Chapter 4 to analyze censored survival data. The rules of the game are essentially the same. First, a comparable "node impurity" is needed in tree growing; that is, we must define a partitioning criterion by which one node is split into two, two into more, and so on. Second, to guide tree pruning, an analogous "cost-complexity" needs to be formulated so that we can choose a "right-sized" tree, or equivalently, determine the terminal nodes. Before discussing these details, we present a tree-based survival analysis in Section 6.2 and reveal the potential of such an analysis in providing new scientific results that are not so readily attainable with other more standard methods.

6.2 Tree-Based Analysis for the Western Collaborative Group Study Data

The Western Collaborative Group Study (WCGS) is a prospective and long-term study of coronary heart disease. In 1960–61, 3,154 middle-aged white males from ten large California corporations in the San Francisco Bay Area and Los Angeles entered the WCGS, and they were free of coronary heart disease and cancer. After a 33-year follow-up, 417 of 1,329 deaths were due to cancer and 43 were lost to follow up. Table 6.1 provides part of the baseline characteristics that were collected from the WCGS. A more detailed description of study design and population is available from Ragland et al. (1988). Table 6.1 gives a brief description of the predictors. In particular, body mass index (BMI) and waist-to-calf ratio (WCR) are two measures of obesity. The question of primary interest here is whether obesity as indicated by BMI and WCR is associated with the risk of cancer.

In classifying binary outcome, the impact of using different splitting criteria is relatively minor. However, the impact appears to be greater for the analysis of censored data. As we will introduce later, several criteria have been studied in the literature. We use two of them in Figure 6.2. One is based on the log-rank statistic and the other from a straightforward extension of node impurities. The next two chapters will provide in-depth discussions, but for the moment, we concentrate on the practical aspect of the analysis.

6.2 Tree-Based Analysis for the Western Collaborative Group Study Data

TABLE 6.1. Eight Selected Baseline Variables from the WCGS

Characteristics	Descriptive Statistics
Age	46.3 ± 5.2 years
Education	High sch. (1,424), Col. (431), Grad. (1298)
Systolic blood pressure	128.6 ± 15.1 mmHg
Serum cholesterol	226.2 ± 42.9 (mg/dl)
Behavior pattern	Type A (1589), type B (1565)
Smoking habits	Yes (2439), No (715) high
Body mass index	24.7 ± 2.7 (kg/m^2)
Waist-to-calf ratio	2.4 ± 0.2

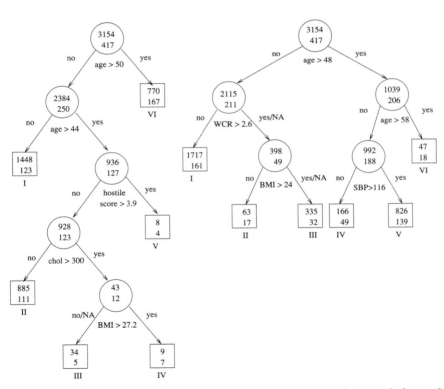

FIGURE 6.2. The survival trees using the log-rank statistic and a straightforward extension of impurity.

76   6. Analysis of Censored Data: Examples

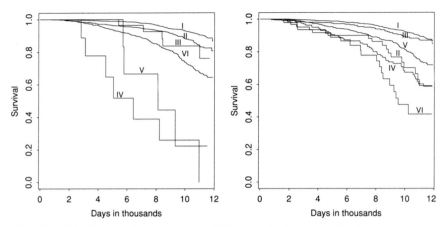

FIGURE 6.3. Kaplan–Meier curves within terminal nodes. The two panels correspond to the two trees in Figure 6.2.

How do we answer the clinical question from the survival trees? A commonly used approach is to draw Kaplan–Meier curves within all terminal nodes and then to compare these curves. Figure 6.3 is prepared following this common wisdom. Thus, the survival trees are employed as a means of stratifying the study sample. This is particularly useful when the proportionality assumption is violated in the Cox model introduced in the next chapter.

Let us first examine the tree on the left of Figure 6.2. As in the proportional hazard model (see Section 7.2.3), age and cholesterol are important attributes to survival. The hostile score seems to matter, but it requires a threshold so high (greater than 3.9) that only 8 subjects crossed the line. Instead of WCR as in the proportional hazard model, BMI, another measure of obesity, expresses some influence on the survival, but is limited to a group of 43 subjects. If we remove three survival curves for the three relatively small nodes, the left panel in Figure 6.3 suggests three major, distinct characteristics of survival, two of which are determined by age (terminal nodes I and VI). The curve for terminal node II shows that lower cholesterol levels have a dramatic protective effect on survival due to cancer.

The six survival curves on the right of Figure 6.3 display four major distinct characteristics of survival. Terminal nodes III and IV deserve our special attention. Let us point out that there are 173 missing values on BMI in terminal node III, of which 18 died from cancer. This death proportion is about the same as that among those who had BMI measured. Although subjects in terminal node I (younger and lower WCR group) had enjoyed the longest survival time, those in terminal node III had a very close survival duration. What is surprising is that this is a group with relatively high WCR and BMI. Based on the survivorship of terminal node II and the discussion above, when only one of WCR and BMI is high, the risk of death

6.2 Tree-Based Analysis for the Western Collaborative Group Study Data

is increased. The survivorship of terminal node V seems to raise another point. For those of age about 50 to 60, moderately high SBP is protective of survival due to cancer. These observations shed some new light on cancer death that was not uncovered from previous analyses. However, the extent of their validity warrants further investigation.

— it is unclear as to whether the outcome is cancer-specific. events add up to 695 not 417!

7
Analysis of Censored Data: Concepts and Classical Methods

Before presenting the methods of survival trees, we should be aware of the methodology in place that is commonly used to analyze censored survival data. It is strategically wise to understand the data and answer scientific questions by different methods and from different perspectives.

7.1 The Basics of Survival Analysis

Survival analysis involves a variety of issues and a thorough coverage is far beyond our scope. Useful textbooks are available at different levels such as Kalbfleisch and Prentice (1980), Miller (1981), and Lee (1992). Here, we focus on basic issues that are relevant to the understanding of survival trees.

Table 7.1 presents the survival time in days along with the smoking history for a random set of 60 subjects from the 1988 Western Collaborative Group Study. We will reanalyze the entire study in Section 7.2.3. What we should notice for the moment is that the censored time is indicated by a plus sign, "+," following the time.

The fundamental question is, How do we describe the survival time of the samples in Table 7.1? This leads to the most basic concept in survival analysis: survival function. It is the probability of surviving longer than a given time. Symbolically, the survival function is defined as

$$S(t) = I\!P\{T > t\}. \qquad (7.1)$$

TABLE 7.1. A Random Sample from the Western Collaborative Group Study

Smoked	Time (days)	Smoked	Time (days)	Smoked	Time (days)
yes	11906+	yes	9389+	yes	4539+
yes	11343+	yes	9515+	yes	10048+
yes	5161	yes	9169	no	8147+
yes	11531+	yes	11403+	yes	11857+
yes	11693+	no	10587	yes	9343+
yes	11293+	yes	6351+	yes	502+
yes	7792	no	11655+	yes	9491+
yes	2482+	no	10773+	yes	11594+
no	7559+	yes	11355+	yes	2397
yes	2569+	yes	2334+	yes	11497+
yes	4882+	yes	9276	yes	703+
yes	10054	no	11875+	no	9946+
yes	11466+	no	10244+	yes	11529+
yes	8757+	no	11467+	yes	4818
yes	7790	yes	11727+	no	9552+
yes	11626+	yes	7887+	yes	11595+
yes	7677+	yes	11503	yes	10396+
yes	6444+	yes	7671+	yes	10529+
yes	11684+	yes	11355+	yes	11334+
yes	10850+	yes	6092	yes	11236+

7.1 The Basics of Survival Analysis

Another concept that is of almost equal importance is the hazard function:

$$h(t) = \frac{\lim_{\Delta t \to 0} \mathbb{P}\{T \in (t, t + \Delta t)\}/\Delta t}{\mathbb{P}\{T > t\}}. \tag{7.2}$$

The hazard function is an instantaneous failure rate in the sense that it measures the chance of an instantaneous failure per unit of time given that an individual has survived beyond time t. Note that the numerator of (7.2) is the density function of T, or the minus derivative of the denominator. Therefore, knowing the survival function is enough to derive the hazard function and vice versa.

The next question is, How do we estimate the survival or hazard function from data such as the samples in Table 7.1 (ignoring the smoking history for the time being)? Two general answers are available to this question. The first one assumes specific knowledge for the distribution of the survival time and hence is parametric, but the second does not and is nonparametric, or distribution-free. We defer the second approach to Section 7.1.1.

For the first approach, different distributions of survival can be assumed. For example, one simple choice is to assume that the survival function is exponential, i.e.,

$$S(t) = \exp(-\lambda t) \ (\lambda > 0), \tag{7.3}$$

where λ is an unknown constant. In fact, λ is the hazard function. Thus, equivalent to (7.3) is that $h(t) = \lambda$, i.e., a constant hazard function. Having made such an assumption, it remains to estimate the only unknown parameter, λ, namely the hazard. This is usually done by maximizing the likelihood function.

When the survival time T_i of individual i is observed, the corresponding density $f(T_i)$ contributes to the likelihood function. When the censoring time U_i is observed, however, the value of the survival function appears in the likelihood function. Thus, the full likelihood function under the assumption (7.3) for the data in Table 7.1 is

$$L(\lambda) = \prod_{i=1}^{60} [\lambda \exp(-\lambda T_i)]^{\delta_i} [\exp(-\lambda U_i)]^{1-\delta_i}, \tag{7.4}$$

the log of which is

$$\begin{aligned} l(\lambda) &= \sum_{i=1}^{60} \{\delta_i[\log(\lambda) - \lambda Y_i] - \lambda(1-\delta_i)Y_i\} \\ &= \log(\lambda) \sum_{i=1}^{60} \delta_i - \lambda \sum_{i=1}^{60} T_i \\ &= 11\log(\lambda) - \lambda(11906 + 11343 + \cdots + 11236), \end{aligned}$$

where 11 is the number of uncensored survival times and the summation is over all observed times. Therefore, the maximum likelihood estimate of the hazard, λ, is

$$\hat{\lambda} = \frac{11}{527240} = 2.05/10^5, \qquad (7.5)$$

which is the number of failures divided by the total observed time; in other words, there were $2.05/10^5$ failures per day. When the hazard function is constant, the estimate in (7.5) follows from the definition.

Assumption (7.3) is one possibility and does not necessarily lead to an adequate fit to the data. Due to censoring, a simple χ^2 goodness-of-fit test is not appropriate. Hollander and Proschan (1979) proposed a formal test making use of the Kaplan–Meier curve described below. In practice, some graphical approaches are more intuitive and easier to appreciate. After presenting the Kaplan–Meier Curve in Section 7.1.1, we can compare a parametric fit with the nonparametric Kaplan–Meier Curve. Another useful approach is hazard plotting (Nelson, 1972), similar to probability plotting. It plots the empirical cumulative hazard function against the assumed theoretical cumulative hazard function at times when failures occurred. Here, the cumulative hazard function is defined as

$$H(t) = \int_0^t h(u)du. \qquad (7.6)$$

Since the hazard is not a density function, the cumulative function may be greater than one. For the exponential survival function, the cumulative hazard function is a linear function: λt.

In Table 7.1 there are 11 time points where deaths occurred. It is easy to obtain the theoretical cumulative hazard function. To calculate the empirical value at time T_i, we first find the number of subjects who survived up to time T_i, denoted by K_i, and then the number of failures at time T_i, denoted by d_i. The hazard rate at T_i is estimated by d_i/K_i, i.e., the ratio of the number of failures to the number of subjects at risk. The cumulative hazard at T_i is the sum of all hazard rates before and at T_i. Table 7.2 displays the process of calculating both empirical and theoretical cumulative hazard functions, where the survival function is assumed to be exponential. The hazard plot in Figure 7.1 implies that the exponential survival is not appropriate for the data, because the empirical and theoretical cumulative hazard functions do not match each other. Therefore, we should refit our survival data by assuming different distributions and then check the goodness of fit. We leave it to interested readers to find appropriate parametric models.

TABLE 7.2. Cumulative Hazard Functions

Survival time	Risk set K	Failures d	Hazard rate d/K	Cumulative hazard Empirical	Cumulative hazard Assumed
2397	57	1	0.0175	0.0175	0.0491
4818	53	1	0.0189	0.0364	0.0988
5161	51	1	0.0196	0.0560	0.1058
6092	50	1	0.0200	0.0760	0.1249
7790	44	1	0.0227	0.0987	0.1597
7792	43	1	0.0233	0.1220	0.1597
9169	39	1	0.0256	0.1476	0.1880
9276	38	1	0.0263	0.1740	0.1902
10054	30	1	0.0333	0.2073	0.2061
10587	26	1	0.0385	0.2458	0.2170
11503	13	1	0.0769	0.3227	0.2358

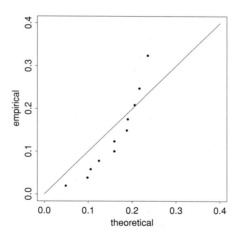

FIGURE 7.1. Cumulative hazard plot

TABLE 7.3. Product Limit Estimate of Survival Function

Survival time	Risk set K	Failures d	Ratio $(K-d)/K$	Product $\hat{S}(t)$
2397	57	1	0.982	0.982
4818	53	1	0.981	$0.982 * 0.981 = 0.963$
5161	51	1	0.980	$0.963 * 0.980 = 0.944$
6092	50	1	0.980	$0.944 * 0.980 = 0.925$
7790	44	1	0.977	$0.925 * 0.977 = 0.904$
7792	43	1	0.977	$0.904 * 0.977 = 0.883$
9169	39	1	0.974	$0.883 * 0.974 = 0.860$
9276	38	1	0.974	$0.860 * 0.974 = 0.838$
10054	30	1	0.967	$0.838 * 0.967 = 0.810$
10587	26	1	0.962	$0.810 * 0.962 = 0.779$
11503	13	1	0.923	$0.779 * 0.923 = 0.719$

7.1.1 Kaplan–Meier Curve

We have shown how to fit survival data with parametric models and have also realized that a particular parametric assumption may not be appropriate for the data. Here, we describe the most commonly used nonparametric method of constructing survival curves, developed by Kaplan and Meier (1958).

The mechanism of producing the Kaplan–Meier curve is similar to the generation of the empirical cumulative hazard function. The first three columns of Table 7.3 are the same as those in Table 7.2. The fourth column in Table 7.3 is one minus the fourth column in Table 7.2, namely, the proportion of individuals who survived beyond the given time point. The last column is a recursive product of the fourth column, giving the product-limit estimate of survival function $\hat{S}(t)$. Figure 7.2 is a plot of $\hat{S}(t)$ against time, the so-called Kaplan–Meier curve.

As mentioned earlier, the Kaplan–Meier curve can also be used to check the adequacy of a parametric survival model. For example, we embedded the exponential survival function into Figure 7.2. It is clear that the exponential survival function underestimates the survival in the early stage and overestimates later. In other words, as also shown by Figure 7.1, the parametric model inflates the hazard rate earlier and shrinks it later. What, then, is the point of using parametric models? When they are appropriate, parametric models can provide a more precise estimate of survival, and their parameters may have clinical interpretation. Miller (1983) examined specific cases where the asymptotic efficiencies of the Kaplan–Meier estimator are low, especially for high censoring proportions.

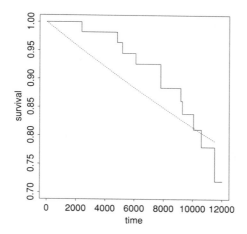

FIGURE 7.2. The Kaplan–Meier (solid) curve and the exponential survival (dotted) curve

7.1.2 Log-Rank Test

In many clinical studies, estimating survival function is the means, not the goal. A common goal is to compare the survival distributions of various groups. For example, we may be interested in whether the survival distributions of the smoking and nonsmoking groups in Table 7.1 differ. As a first step, we may view the Kaplan–Meier curves graphically, as illustrated in Figure 7.3. The short vertical lines along the survival curves in this figure mark the censoring times. The two curves appear to be different. In particular, the nonsmokers seem to have survived longer. Note, however, that Table 7.1 contains a small fraction of the Western Collaborative Group Study. Hence, the clinical conclusions drawn here are for the purpose of illustrating the method. A complete analysis will be conducted later.

Although graphical presentations are useful, it is also important to test the significance of the difference in the survival distributions. Many test statistics have been developed and studied in depth. Among them is Mantel's log-rank test, generalized from Savage's (1956) test. The name of the log-rank test was given by Peto and Peto (1972).

At the distinct failure times, we have a sequence of 2×2 tables

	Dead	Alive	
Smoking	a_i		n_i
Nonsmoking			
	d_i		K_i

86   7. Analysis of Censored Data: Concepts and Classical Methods

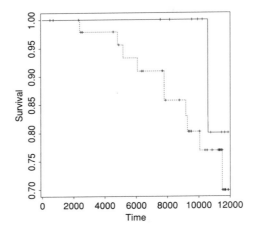

FIGURE 7.3. The Kaplan–Meier curves for smoking (dotted) and nonsmoking groups (solid)

TABLE 7.4. Calculation of Log-Rank Test

Time T_i	Risk set K_i	Failures d_i	a_i	n_i	E_i	V_i
2397	57	1	1	47	0.825	0.145
4818	53	1	1	43	0.811	0.153
5161	51	1	1	41	0.804	0.158
6092	50	1	1	40	0.800	0.160
7790	44	1	1	35	0.795	0.163
7792	43	1	1	34	0.791	0.165
9169	39	1	1	31	0.795	0.163
9276	38	1	1	30	0.789	0.166
10054	30	1	1	24	0.800	0.160
10587	26	1	0	21	0.808	0.155
11503	13	1	1	11	0.846	0.130

For the data in Table 7.1, the counts of a_i, d_i, n_i, and K_i are calculated in Table 7.4. The log-rank test statistic is

$$LR = \frac{\sum_{i=1}^{k}(a_i - E_i)}{\sqrt{\sum_{i=1}^{k} V_i}}, \qquad (7.7)$$

where k is the number of distinct failure times,

$$E_i = \frac{d_i n_i}{K_i},$$

and

$$V_i = \left(\frac{d_i(K_i - n_i)n_i}{K_i(K_i - 1)}\right)\left(1 - \frac{d_i}{K_i}\right).$$

Since the log-rank test statistic has an asymptotic standard normal distribution, we test the hypothesis that the two survival functions are the same by comparing LR with the quantiles of the standard normal distribution. For our data, $LR = 0.87$, corresponding to a two-sided p-value of 0.38.

7.2 Parametric Regression for Censored Data

What we have discussed so far is only enough to deal with simple issues such as the comparison of two survival functions. In most applications, however, the question of interest is more challenging. In Examples 6.1–6.3, we have seen that the determinants of survival are multifactorial. How, then, do we establish the relationship between survival and a number of covariates? We present two approaches to answering this question. The first one is intuitively appealing, but not quite successful.

7.2.1 Linear Regression with Censored Data*

Consider the simple linear regression model

$$Y_i = \alpha + \beta x_i + \epsilon_i,$$

for n pairs of observations (x_i, Y_i) $(i = 1, \ldots, n)$. In the absence of censoring, it is standard to estimate the regression coefficients through the least squares criterion. That is, the estimates $\hat{\alpha}$ and $\hat{\beta}$ are those values of α and β that minimize the sum of squares

$$\sum_{i=1}^{n}(Y_i - \alpha - \beta x_i)^2 = n\int z^2 d\hat{F}(z;\alpha,\beta), \qquad (7.8)$$

where $\hat{F}(z;\alpha,\beta)$ is the empirical distribution of $Y_i - \alpha - \beta x_i$ $(i = 1, \ldots, n)$.

In the censored case, Miller (1976) proposed to replace $\hat{F}(z; \alpha, \beta)$ in (7.8) with the Kaplan–Meier estimate. This proposal is conceptually simple, but it has two serious shortcomings: (a) The analytic properties of the resulting estimates $\hat{\alpha}$ and $\hat{\beta}$ are difficult to study because the minimum of (7.8) can occur at a discontinuity point. In fact, the estimates are, in general, inconsistent (Buckley and James, 1979). (b) The method faces computational obstacles in multiple regression because the occurrence of minima at discontinuous points makes it necessary to have a grid search for the estimates.

To overcome the problems with Miller's method and stay in the domain of the standard linear regression, Buckley and James (1979) suggested a different idea. For a censored time, we have $U_i < T_i$. If we knew the difference $T_i - U_i$, we could add it to our observed time Y_i. After this, we would not have censored data, and the standard methodology would be applicable. Obviously, we do not know the difference. Their first step is to replace the difference by the conditional mean difference $E(T_i - U_i | T_i > U_i)$. In other words, the observations become

$$Y_i^* = Y_i \delta_i + E(T_i | T_i > Y_i)(1 - \delta_i) \ (i = 1, \ldots, n).$$

It is important to observe that $E(Y_i^*) = \alpha + \beta x_i$ when the linear model holds for the underlying survival time. It follows that

$$E\left[\sum_{i=1}^{n}(x_i - \bar{x})(Y_i^* - \beta x_i)\right] = 0,$$

which is analogous to the normal equations in the standard linear regression. Because of this fact, Buckley and James chose the slope estimate $\hat{\beta}$ such that

$$\sum_{i=1}^{n}(x_i - \bar{x})(Y_i^* - \hat{\beta} x_i) = 0.$$

This type of estimate is called an M-estimate in the context of robust statistics (e.g., Huber, 1981).

Unfortunately, Y_i^* is still not available from the data. In the second step, Buckley and James adopted a self-consistent approach to approximate Y_i^* for censored individuals. On average, it is βx_i. Given that we observed a censoring time U_i, what is a reasonable estimate of $\Delta_i = Y_i^* - \beta x_i$? To find the answer, consider the adjusted time $Z_i = Y_i - \beta x_i \ (i = 1, \ldots, n)$. We can find the Kaplan–Meier estimate $\hat{S}(z)$ for the adjusted time Z_i. Now, Δ_i can be estimated by a weighted average of Z_k among those uncensored individuals for whom $Z_k > \Delta_i$, i.e., those who survived beyond Δ_i under the adjusted time scale. More precisely,

$$\tilde{\Delta}_i = \sum_{\{k: \delta_k = 1, Z_k > \Delta_k\}} \frac{v(Z_k)}{\hat{S}(Z_k)} Z_k,$$

where $v(Z_k) = \lim_{\Delta \to 0} S(Z_k - \Delta) - S(Z_k)$. Then, we use

$$\tilde{Y}_i(\beta) = \beta x_i + \tilde{\Delta}_i$$

to replace the censoring time. Such a replacement leads to an estimator $\tilde{\beta}$ that satisfies

$$\tilde{\beta} = \frac{\sum_{i=1}^n (x_i - \bar{x})[Y_i \delta_i + \tilde{Y}_i(\beta)(1 - \delta_i)]}{\sum_{i=1}^n (x_i - \bar{x})^2}. \tag{7.9}$$

Since both sides of (7.9) depend on β, the solution needs to be found by an iterative algorithm. Unfortunately, an exact solution is not guaranteed. When no solution exists, Buckley and James found that the iterations usually settle down to oscillating between two values. Once a slope $\tilde{\beta}$ is chosen, the corresponding estimate $\tilde{\alpha}$ of the intercept is

$$\tilde{\alpha} = \frac{1}{n} \sum_{i=1}^n [Y_i \delta_i + \tilde{Y}_i(\beta)(1 - \delta_i)] - \tilde{\beta} \bar{x}.$$

Since a unique solution is not guaranteed, the properties of the estimates are also difficult to study. We described these unsuccessful attempts because they could otherwise lead to an easy extension of the tree-based method for the analysis of censored data. In that case, we could attach a patch to any censored time and use it as if it were a survival time.

7.2.2 Cox Proportional Hazard Regression

Instead of making assumptions directly on the survival times, Cox (1972) proposed to specify the hazard function. As before, suppose that we have a set of predictors $\mathbf{x} = (x_1, \ldots, x_p)$ in addition to our survival time. The Cox proportional hazard model assumes that

$$\lambda(t; \mathbf{x}) = \exp(\mathbf{x}\boldsymbol{\beta})\lambda_0(t), \tag{7.10}$$

where $\boldsymbol{\beta}$ is a $p \times 1$ vector of unknown parameters and $\lambda_0(t)$ is an unknown function giving a baseline hazard for $\mathbf{x} = \mathbf{0}$. As a trivial note, the part $\mathbf{x}\boldsymbol{\beta}$ can be extended to a general function in $\mathbf{x}$. The unique feature of (7.10) is that if we take two individuals i and j with covariates $\mathbf{x}_i$ and $\mathbf{x}_j$, the ratio of their hazard functions is $\exp((\mathbf{x}_i - \mathbf{x}_j)\boldsymbol{\beta})$, which is free of time. In other words, the hazard functions for any two individuals are parallel in time. It is critical to keep in mind this fact when we validate the assumption (7.10) in applications.

Note that $\lambda_0(t)$ is left to be arbitrary in (7.10). Thus, the proportional hazard can be regarded as semiparametric. To estimate $\boldsymbol{\beta}$, Cox suggested using a conditional likelihood without estimating the nuisance $\lambda_0(t)$. He argued that no information can be contributed about $\boldsymbol{\beta}$ by time intervals

90   7. Analysis of Censored Data: Concepts and Classical Methods

in which no failures occur, because the component $\lambda_0(t)$ might be zero in such intervals. Therefore, the likelihood should be conditioned on the set of uncensored times.

At any time t, let $\mathcal{R}(t)$ be the risk set, i.e., the individuals who were at risk right before time t. For each uncensored time T_i, the hazard rate is

$$h(T_i) = I\!\!P\{\text{A death in } (T_i, T_i + dt) \mid \mathcal{R}(T_i)\}/dt.$$

Hence, under the proportion hazard model,

$$I\!\!P\{\text{A death in } (T_i, T_i + dt) \mid \mathcal{R}(T_i)\} = \exp(\mathbf{x}\boldsymbol{\beta})\lambda_0(T_i)dt$$

and

$$I\!\!P\{\text{Individual } i \text{ fails at } T_i \mid \text{one death in } \mathcal{R}(T_i) \text{ at time } T_i\}$$
$$= \frac{\exp(\mathbf{x}_i\boldsymbol{\beta})}{\sum_{j \in \mathcal{R}(T_i)} \exp(\mathbf{x}_j\boldsymbol{\beta})}.$$

The conditional probability above is the contribution of failed individual i to the conditional likelihood and altogether the conditional likelihood is the product

$$L(\boldsymbol{\beta}) = \prod_{\text{failure } i} \frac{\exp(\mathbf{x}_i\boldsymbol{\beta})}{\sum_{j \in \mathcal{R}(T_i)} \exp(\mathbf{x}_j\boldsymbol{\beta})}. \qquad (7.11)$$

Maximizing the conditional likelihood (7.11) gives rise to the estimates of $\boldsymbol{\beta}$. Like the ordinary maximum likelihood estimates, $\hat{\boldsymbol{\beta}}$ has an asymptotic normal distribution. We refer the detailed theory to Fleming and Harrington (1991).

To further justify the use of the conditional likelihood (7.11), Kalbfleisch and Prentice (1973) showed that (7.11) is also the joint probability of the ranks of the observed times as compared to the uncensored times only. More precisely, define

$$R_i = \begin{cases} \text{rank of } Y_i \text{ among uncensored times} & \text{if } \delta_i = 1, \\ \text{rank of the preceding uncensored time} & \text{if } \delta_i = 0. \end{cases}$$

Then the joint probability distribution of (R_i, δ_i) $(i = 1, \ldots, n)$ equals (7.11).

Once $\hat{\boldsymbol{\beta}}$ is available, there is a variety of ways to estimate the baseline hazard $\lambda_0(t)$. The entire model estimation and validation procedure has been implemented in standard software such as the coxph and cox.zph functions in SPLUS. See S-PLUS guide (1995).

TABLE 7.5. Parameter Estimation for Cox's Model

Variable	Coefficient	S.E.	p-value
Age (age)	0.0934	0.009	0.000
Serum cholesterol (chol)	0.0026	0.001	0.033
Smoking habits (smoke)	0.2263	0.103	0.029
Waist-to-calf ratio (wcr)	0.7395	0.271	0.006

7.2.3 Reanalysis of the Western Collaborative Group Study Data

We entered the eight predictors in Table 6.1 into an initial Cox's model and used a backward stepwise procedure to delete the least significant variable from the model at the threshold of 0.05. Table 6.1 gives a brief description of the predictors. In particular, body-mass index (BMI) and waist-to-calf ratio (WCR) are two measures of obesity. Due to the missing values of education, BMI and WCR, 277 subjects were removed first in the model selection. After three steps, we deleted education from the model, and 277 subjects still had missing values on BMI and WCR. After one more step, we removed BMI from the model and then added back into the model selection 5 subjects whose WCR's were complete. The computation was carried out in SPLUS, and the final model was built by the function

coxph(Surv(time, cancer)~age + chol + smoke + wcr).

The estimates of the coefficients, their standard errors, and p-values are reported in Table 7.5.

Before we finish with Cox's model, we must assess the proportional hazard assumption. To this end, we use both a graphical approach and a theoretical approach developed by Grambsch and Therneau (1994).

To use the graphical approach, we dichotomize age, serum cholesterol, and waist-to-calf ratio at their median levels. Then, the 2882 (= 3154−272) subjects are divided into 16 cohorts. Within each cohort i, we calculate the Kaplan–Meier survival estimate $\hat{S}_i(t)$. Next, we plot $\log(-\log(\hat{S}_i(t)))$ versus time as shown in Figure 7.4. In each of the four panels, four curves are displayed.

Now, how do we assess the proportional hazard assumption on the basis of Figure 7.4? It follows from the definition of hazard function in (7.2) that

$$h(t) = -\frac{d\log(S(t))}{dt},$$

which is equivalent to

$$S(t) = \exp\left(-\int_0^t h(z)dz\right).$$

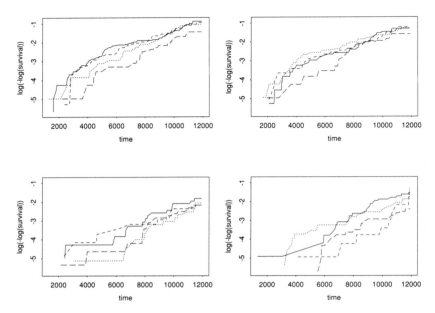

FIGURE 7.4. Log-log Kaplan–Meier curves for 16 cohorts

According to (7.10), the survival function is

$$S(t; \mathbf{x}) = \exp\left[-\int_0^t \exp(\mathbf{x}\boldsymbol{\beta})\lambda_0(z)\right]$$
$$= \exp\left[-\exp(\mathbf{x}\boldsymbol{\beta})\int_0^t \lambda_0(z)\right]. \quad (7.12)$$

In other words,

$$\log(-\log[S(t; \mathbf{x})]) = \mathbf{x}\boldsymbol{\beta} + \log\left[\int_0^t \lambda_0(z)\right]. \quad (7.13)$$

As a consequence, the log-log survival curves in our 16 cohorts are supposed to be parallel if the proportion hazard assumption holds. Figure 7.4 does not suggest any clear violation of the assumption, although some crossover of curves can be identified in the bottom-right panel.

Using the SPLUS function cox.zph to test whether the assumption is met in the statistical sense, the global p-value is 0.3. However, there may be some marginal violation with respect to age for which the p-value is 0.04. In summary, the proportion hazard model appears reasonable to the WCGS data.

In summary, Table 7.5 suggests that age, high serum cholesterol level, smoking, and obesity have negative effects on survival. This is obviously an old story that has been repeated by many epidemiologic and experimental studies.

8
Analysis of Censored Data: Survival Trees

We elucidated in Chapter 4 the usefulness of the recursive partitioning technique for the analysis of binary outcomes. Not only can this technique be extended to the analysis of censored data, but also, as pointed out by Gordon and Olshen (1985), tree-based regression is applicable to more general situations than that of the proportion hazard regression described previously. As a matter of fact, the most popular use of the tree-based methods is in the area of survival analysis.

8.1 Splitting Criteria

Several splitting criteria have been developed since the publication of the CART book of Breiman et al. (1984). We describe them in chronological order. Although the relative merits of these criteria are not clearly resolved, it seems safe for users to begin with the use of the log-rank statistic. In many applications, it is useful to generate trees from different criteria and select one of them based on scientific judgment. In this sense, a theoretical settlement of one criterion being superior to others is less important.

8.1.1 Gordon and Olshen's Rule*

Gordon and Olshen (1985) made the first attempt to adapt the idea of recursive partitioning to cover censored survival analysis. When classifying binary outcomes in Section 4.1, we introduced the concept of node impurity.

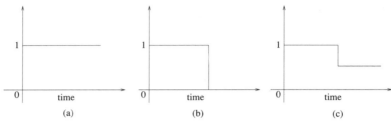

FIGURE 8.1. Three possible Kaplan–Meier curves for a homogeneous node. (a) All observations were censored; (b) All failures occurred at the same time and there was no censored observation afterwards; (c) All failures occurred at the same time, followed by censored times.

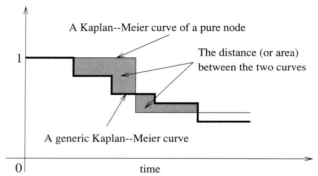

FIGURE 8.2. The L^1 Wasserstein distance between two Kaplan–Meier curves

What would be an appropriate measure of node impurity in the context of censored data? We would regard a node as pure if all failures in the node occurred at the same time. In such circumstances, the shape of the Kaplan–Meier curve within the node has three possibilities, as depicted in Figure 8.1. In other words, the curve has at most one drop. Let $\mathcal{P}$ be the collection of all such Kaplan–Meier curves.

One way to judge the node impurity is to see how far the within-node Kaplan–Meier curve deviates from any of the curves in $\mathcal{P}$. To this end, we need first to define a distance between the two Kaplan–Meier curves. Gordon and Olshen used the so-called L^p Wasserstein metrics $d_p(\cdot, \cdot)$ as the measure of discrepancy between the two survival functions. Graphically, when $p = 1$, the Wasserstein distance $d_1(S_1, S_2)$ between two Kaplan–Meier curves S_1 and S_2 is the shaded area in Figure 8.2. In general, $d_p(\cdot, \cdot)$ is defined as follows.

8.1 Splitting Criteria

Let F_1 and F_2 be two distribution functions. The L^p Wasserstein distance between F_1 and F_2 is

$$\left[\int_0^1 |F_1^{-1}(u) - F_2^{-1}(u)|^p du\right]^{1/p}, \tag{8.1}$$

where $F_i^{-1}(u) = \min\{t : F_i(t) \geq u\}, i = 1, 2$.

Now, let us take $F_1(t) = 1 - S_1(t)$ and $F_2(t) = 1 - S_2(t)$. Note that F_1 and F_2 have all the properties of a distribution function except that they may not approach 1 at the right end, which occurs when the longest observed time is censored; see, e.g., Figure 8.1(a, c). Formally,

$$\lim_{t\to\infty} F_1(t) = m_1 \leq 1 \text{ and } \lim_{t\to\infty} F_2(t) = m_2 \leq 1.$$

Such F_1 and F_2 are called improper distribution functions. If we can generalize the distance metrics in (8.1) to improper distribution functions, then we can define the distance between two Kaplan–Meier curves as that between the respectively flipped improper distribution functions. Indeed, the L^p Wasserstein distance between S_1 and S_2 can be defined as

$$\left[\int_0^m |F_1^{-1}(u) - F_2^{-1}(u)|^p du\right]^{1/p}, \tag{8.2}$$

where the upper limit of the integral m is the minimum of m_1 and m_2. To avoid technicalities, this definition is slightly simpler than the original version of Gordon and Olshen.

We are ready now to define the node impurity. If a node is pure, the corresponding Kaplan–Meier curve should be one of the three curves in Figure 8.1. Otherwise, we can compare the within-node Kaplan–Meier curve with the three forms of curves in Figure 8.1. These comparisons reveal the degree of node purity. In formal terms, the impurity of node τ is defined as

$$i(\tau) = \min_{\delta_S \in \mathcal{P}} d_p(S_\tau, \delta_S), \tag{8.3}$$

where S_τ is the Kaplan–Meier curve within node τ, and the minimization $\min_{\delta_S \in \mathcal{P}}$ means that S_τ is compared with its best match among the curves of the forms depicted in Figure 8.1.

In general, the numerical implementation of (8.3) is not a straightforward task, although it is clear in a theoretical sense thanks to the fact that the distance is a convex function. When $p = 1$, the impurity in (8.3) can be viewed as the deviation of survival times toward their median. When $p = 2$, the impurity in (8.3) corresponds to the variance of the Kaplan–Meier distribution estimate of survival. Other than the theoretical generality, there is no loss for us to choose p equal to either 1 or 2.

After the preparation above, we can divide a node into two as follows. First, we compute the Kaplan–Meier curves as in Section 7.1.1 separately for each daughter node. Then, we calculate the node impurities from (8.3). A desirable split can be characterized as the one that results in the smallest weighted impurity. This selection procedure is identical to that discussed in Section 2.2. Indeed, we use (2.3) again to select a split; namely, the goodness of a split s is

$$\Delta I(s,\tau) = i(\tau) - I\!P\{\tau_L\}i(\tau_L) - I\!P\{\tau_R\}i(\tau_R). \qquad (8.4)$$

Once a node is partitioned into two, we can continue to partition recursively as in the classification of binary outcome and eventually reach an initially large tree. The pruning of a large survival tree is the topic of Section 8.2.

8.1.2 Maximizing the Difference

Using the distance between two Kaplan–Meier curves, we can split a node with an alternative measure. Heuristically, when two daughter nodes are relatively pure, they tend to differ from each other. In other words, if one split gives rise to two different-looking daughter nodes, each of them is likely to be relatively homogeneous. It is perhaps easier to think about the situation in the analysis of variance table where the larger the between variation is, the smaller the within variation is. Finding two different daughters is a means to increase the between variation and consequently to reduce the within variation. The latter implies the homogeneity of the two daughter nodes. If we take this point of view, we then select a split that maximizes the "difference" between the two daughter nodes, or, equivalently, minimizes their similarity. For example, we may select a split such that $d_1(S_L, S_R)$ is maximized; here S_L and S_R are the Kaplan–Meier curves of the left and right daughter nodes. Unfortunately, some empirical evidence appears to suggest that this idea does not perform as well as the other splitting criteria do.

As we discussed in Section 7.1.2, the log-rank test is a commonly used approach for testing the significance of the difference between the survival times of two groups. Motivated by this fact, Ciampi et al. (1986) and Segal (1988) suggested selecting a split that results in the largest log-rank test statistic. Although not extensive, numerical evidence indicates that the log-rank test is a satisfactory dissimilarity criterion in the construction of survival trees.

8.1.3 Use of Likelihood Functions*

Several likelihood-based splitting criteria have also been proposed in the literature. Davis and Anderson (1989) assume that the survival function within any given node is an exponential function with a constant hazard, as given in (7.3). Within each node, the likelihood function can be easily obtained as in (7.4). Under their assumption, the maximum of the log likelihood in node τ is

$$l(\tau) = \sum_{i \in \tau} \delta_i [\log(\hat{\lambda}_\tau) - 1], \tag{8.5}$$

where $\hat{\lambda}_\tau$ is the hazard estimate. They select the split that maximizes $l(\tau_L) + l(\tau_R)$; here τ_L and τ_R are two daughter nodes.

The splitting criterion of LeBlanc and Crowley (1992) and Ciampi et al. (1995) are both based on the assumption that the hazard functions in two daughter nodes are proportional, but unknown. The difference between their two approaches is whether the full or partial likelihood function in the Cox proportional hazard model should be used. Here, we describe only how to make use of the full likelihood and introduce a splitting rule that is slightly simpler than that of LeBlanc and Crowley (1992) at a conceptual level.

We shall see shortly that the use of likelihood generated from the Cox model as the basis of splitting requires much more in-depth understanding of survival concepts than does that of the log-rank test. On the other hand, LeBlanc and Crowley (1992) acknowledged that their simulation studies suggested similar performance between the two approaches. Therefore, those who are interested basically in the practical use of survival trees may choose to skip the following discussion. From a methodological point of view, it is useful to know how parametric ideas can be adopted in the nonparametric framework.

Assuming the proportional hazard model, all individuals in node τ have the hazard

$$\lambda_\tau(t) = \theta_\tau \lambda_0(t), \tag{8.6}$$

where $\lambda_0(t)$ is the baseline hazard independent of the node and θ_τ is a nonnegative parameter corresponding to $\exp(\mathbf{x}\boldsymbol{\beta})$ in (7.10). Recall that at the time of splitting we use one covariate at a time and treat the value of that covariate as the same inside each daughter node. This is why $\exp(\mathbf{x}\boldsymbol{\beta})$ becomes a single parameter θ_τ in (8.6).

Based on (8.6) and following (7.12), the survival function of individuals in node τ is

$$S(t; \tau) = \exp[-\theta_\tau \Lambda_0(t)], \tag{8.7}$$

where $\Lambda_0(t)$ is the baseline cumulative hazard function integrated from $\lambda_0(t)$.

Using the same argument that led to the full likelihood in (7.4), we have the full likelihood function within node τ as

$$L(\theta_\tau, \lambda_0) = \prod_{\{i \in \text{ node } \tau\}} [\lambda_0(T_i)\theta_\tau]^{\delta_i} \exp[-\Lambda_0(U_i)\theta_\tau]. \tag{8.8}$$

Then, the full likelihood of the entire learning sample for a tree $\mathcal{T}$ can be expressed as

$$L(\boldsymbol{\theta}, \lambda_0; \mathcal{T}) = \prod_{\tau \in \tilde{\mathcal{T}}} L(\theta_\tau, \lambda_0), \qquad (8.9)$$

which is the product of the full likelihoods contributed by all terminal nodes of $\mathcal{T}$.

Every time we partition a node into two, we need to maximize the full tree likelihood (8.9). It is immediately clear that this would be too ambitious for computation, because maximizing (8.9) is usually impractical. Even worse is the fact that the cumulative hazard Λ_0 is unknown in practice, and it must be estimated over and over again, since it is shared by all nodes. Given the potential number of splits we have to go through, it is obviously computationally prohibitive to pursue the precise solution. Furthermore, due to the overall role of Λ_0, it is not apparent that we would arrive at the same tree structure if we split the nodes in different orders. For example, after the root node is divided, we may split the left daughter node first and then the right one, and we may reverse the order. It is desirable that this order has no consequence on the tree structure. As a remedy, LeBlanc and Crowley propose to use a one-step Breslow's (1972) estimate:

$$\hat{\Lambda}_0(t) = \frac{\sum_{i:Y_i \leq t} \delta_i}{|\mathcal{R}(t)|}, \qquad (8.10)$$

where the denominator $|\mathcal{R}(t)|$ is the number of subjects at risk at time t. Hence, it is simply the Nelson (1969) cumulative hazard estimator; see Table 7.2. The one-step estimate of θ_τ is then

$$\hat{\theta}_\tau = \frac{\sum_{\{i \in \text{ node } \tau\}} \delta_i}{\sum_{\{i \in \text{ node } \tau\}} \hat{\Lambda}_0(Y_i)}, \qquad (8.11)$$

which can be interpreted as the number of failures divided by the expected number of failures in node τ under the assumption of no structure in survival times.

LeBlanc and Crowley (1992) suggest splitting a node on the basis of deviance within each of the daughter nodes. To avoid the introduction of deviance, we prefer splitting a node without it. Recall at the end of Section 2.2 that the entropy node impurity is proportional to the maximum of the log likelihood function under the binomial distribution. Thus, we maximize the "likelihood" function (8.9) by substituting θ with (8.11) and λ_0 with

$$\hat{\lambda}_0(Y_i) = \frac{\delta_i}{|\mathcal{R}(t)|},$$

which follows from (8.10).

Note that $\hat{\lambda}_0(Y_i)$ can be estimated before the splitting. If we were to split node τ into nodes τ_L and τ_R, we would maximize the sum of the log likelihoods from the two daughter nodes; that is,

$$\sum_{i \in \tau_L} \{\delta_i \log[\hat{\lambda}_0(Y_i)\hat{\theta}_{\tau_L}] - \hat{\Lambda}_0(t)\hat{\theta}_{\tau_L}\} + \sum_{i \in \tau_R} \{\delta_i \log[\hat{\lambda}_0(Y_i)\hat{\theta}_{\tau_R}] - \hat{\Lambda}_0(t)\hat{\theta}_{\tau_R}\}.$$

In contrast, if the deviance measure were used, we would need only to replace $\hat{\lambda}_0$ in the expressed above with $\hat{\Lambda}_0$.

8.1.4 A Straightforward Extension

All splitting rules except that of Davis and Anderson (1989) are relatively complicated, particularly to those who are unfamiliar with survival analysis. Are there any simple methods that are potentially useful? In Section 7.2.1, we made an attempt to create "complete" observations for the censored times. If successful, we may use the regression trees of Breiman et al. (1984) without any modification. Unfortunately, the adding-back process is complicated and does not possess desirable properties.

Zhang (1995a) examined a straightforward tree-based approach to censored survival data. Note that we observe a binary death indicator, δ, and the observed time. If we regard them as two outcomes, we can compute the within-node impurity, i_δ, of the death indicator and the within-node quadratic loss function, i_y, of the time. For example, $i_\delta(\tau)$ can be chosen as the entropy in (4.4) and $i_y(\tau)$ as the variance of Y_i in node τ standardized by the variance in the learning sample (or optionally the parent node). Alternatively, perhaps more reasonably, we can exclude censored survival times while deriving $i_y(\tau)$. Then, the within-node impurity for both the death indicator and the time is a weighted combination: $w_\delta i_\delta + w_y i_y$. Zhang (1995a) explored the effect of various weights w_δ and w_y and found the equal weights (1:1) to be a reasonable choice.

One would naturally be skeptical regarding the performance of such a splitting rule. Several applications to real data, including Section 6.2, have indicated that this approach is a fruitful alternative. Perhaps surprisingly, a preliminary simulation (Zhang, 1995a) suggested that this simple extension outperforms the more sophisticated ones in discovering the underlying structures of data. More extensive simulations are warranted, though.

8.2 Pruning a Survival Tree

Using any of the splitting criteria above, we can produce an initial tree. The next issue is obviously, How do we prune the initial survival tree, $\mathcal{T}$? Recall the discussion in Section 2.3; the key element in pruning is the introduction of cost-complexity. In (4.7), we defined the cost-complexity of tree $\mathcal{T}$ as

$$R_\alpha(\mathcal{T}) = R(\mathcal{T}) + \alpha|\tilde{\mathcal{T}}|, \tag{8.12}$$

where $R(\mathcal{T})$ is the sum of the costs over all terminal nodes of $\mathcal{T}$. It is clear that the remaining steps are identical to those in Section 4.2.3 if we can define an appropriate node cost $R(\tau)$ for survival trees.

While proposing their splitting criteria, most authors have also suggested pruning rules that are closely related to the splitting principles. For instance, Gordon and Olshen (1985) suggested using the impurity (8.3) also as the node cost, $R(\tau)$. Davis and Anderson (1989) take $-l(\tau)$ in (8.5) as $R(\tau)$. The truth of the matter is that the splitting and pruning rules do not have to be directly related. In practice, as long as it is appropriate, one should feel free to match a splitting rule with any of the pruning rules. It would be a useful project to scrutinize whether there exists a robust match that results in satisfactory fits to censored data in a variety of settings.

Akin to the cost-complexity, LeBlanc and Crowley (1993) introduced the notion of split-complexity as a substitute for cost-complexity in pruning a survival tree. Let $LR(\tau)$ be the value of the log-rank test at node τ. Then the split-complexity measure is

$$LR_\alpha(\mathcal{T}) = \sum_{\tau \notin \tilde{\mathcal{T}}} LR(\tau) - \alpha(|\tilde{\mathcal{T}}| - 1).$$

Note that the summation above is over the set of internal (nonterminal) nodes and $|\tilde{\mathcal{T}}| - 1$ is the number of internal nodes. The negative sign in front of α is a reflection of the fact that LR_α is to be maximized, whereas the cost-complexity R_α is minimized. LeBlanc and Crowley recommend choosing α between 2 and 4 if the log-rank test is expressed in the χ_1^2 form. A penalty of 4 corresponds roughly to the 0.05 significance level for a split, and that of 2 is consistent with the use of AIC (Akaike 1974). As is the case in the classification of binary outcome (see, e.g., Section 4.6), the log-rank test statistic is usually over optimistic for each split, due to the split selection. LeBlanc and Crowley used bootstrap techniques to deflate the value of LR.

In addition, Segal (1988) recommended a practical bottom-up procedure. This procedure was described in the context of classifying a dichotomous outcome in Section 4.5, except that now the χ^2 statistic should be replaced with the log-rank test statistic (7.7). We will go through this procedure with real data in Section 8.4.

8.3 Implementation

The implementation of survival trees is more complicated than that of classification trees. The calculation of the Kaplan–Meier curves, log-rank

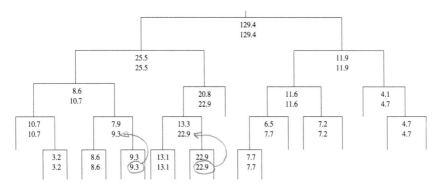

FIGURE 8.3. An initial large tree obtained by the log-rank testing statistic. The top and bottom numbers under the node are respectively the original and maximized values of the statistic.

statistics, or likelihood functions is not an easy task if it has to be repeated a large number of times. It is prudent to achieve the greatest computational efficiency.

As was shown by the data presented in Table 7.4, whether to calculate the within-node Kaplan–Meier curve or to conduct a two-node log-rank test, we need to compute four key quantities, K_i, d_i, a_i, and n_i, which were defined in Section 7.1.2. Obviously, we want efficient algorithms for updating these quantities while searching for the best node split. For instance, let $K_i(\tau)$ be the number of individuals at risk at time t_i within node τ. We consider splitting τ into τ_L and τ_R, say, based on BMI. To make the matter simpler, suppose that BMI takes only three distinct levels in our data: 24, 26, and 28. First, we should obtain K_i at each level of BMI and label them as K_i^{24}, K_i^{26}, and K_i^{28}. Then, the first allowable split is to let the individuals with BMI of 24 be contained in τ_L and the rest in τ_R. It is clear that $K_i(\tau_L) = K_i^{24}$ and $K_i(\tau_R) = K_i^{26} + K_i^{28}$. For the next allowable split, we add K_i^{26} to $K_i(\tau_L)$, whereas $K_i(\tau_R)$ is reduced by K_i^{26}. This goes on until we run out all of allowable splits. The point here is that we should count K_i's once for every level of the predictor and use them subsequently in the splitting.

8.4 Survival Trees for the Western Collaborative Group Study Data

In Section 6.2 we showed how to draw conclusions from survival trees. Here, we provide the details for the construction of the trees in Figure 6.2. This helps us gain insight into the actual process of survival tree generation.

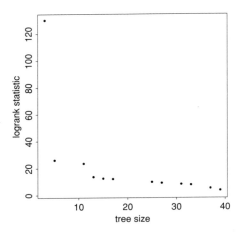

FIGURE 8.4. Maximum log-rank statistic vs. tree size

Let us first use the log-rank test statistic as the basis of node splitting. Figure 8.3 presents the profile of an initial tree with 39 nodes. The original (top) and maximized (bottom) values of the log-rank test statistic are given for each node split. As explained in Section 4.5, the maximized value of the statistic is the maximum of all log-rank test statistics over the subtree rooted at the node of focus. Obviously, the original and maximized log-rank test statistics are identical for all terminal nodes. If we take the root node as an example, both the original and maximized log-rank test statistics are 129.4, because 129.4 is the maximum statistic over the entire tree.

Although we can prune the tree in Figure 8.3 using cross-validation based on the measure of cost-complexity or split-complexity, we decided here to use the alternative pruning method. The reason for this decision is that we can actually get our hands on the steps involved in the pruning process. In Figure 8.4, we plot the maximum log-rank test statistics against the tree size. The tree size in the plot is determined by taking one of the maximum statistics as the threshold and then pruning off all offspring of an internal node whose the maximum log-rank test statistic is below the threshold. What we want to look for in such a plot is a "kink" in the trend. Although this is an unguaranteed, subjective process, it seems to work fine in practice, provided that we use it with caution. After viewing the scatter plot in Figure 8.4, we chose the final tree with 13 nodes, as illustrated on the left-hand side of Figure 6.2.   p. 75.

For comparison, we also grow trees using another splitting criterion. In particular, on the right-hand side of Figure 6.2 we displayed a tree derived from the use of the combined impurity $w_\delta i_\delta + w_y i_y$. It is important to point out here that data analysts do not have to take the computer output as it stands. Reasonable and justifiable changes can be made. To emphasize

8.4 Survival Trees for the Western Collaborative Group Study Data

this point, let use explain what we did before the construction of the tree in the right panel of Figure 6.2. At first, we arrived at a tree with 7 nodes by reviewing an analogous scatter plot to Figure 8.4. If we had taken that 7-node tree, the right daughter node of the root node would have been a terminal node. To make the tree compatible in size to the one on the left of Figure 6.2, we sought to partition the right daughter node of the root node by lowering the pruning threshold of the maximum log-rank statistic within an internal node. This, however, results in a tree that was slightly larger than what we wanted. As a remedy, we pruned off two internal nodes because their maximum log-rank statistics are relatively small.

9
Regression Trees and Adaptive Splines for a Continuous Response

The theme of this chapter is to model the relationship between a continuous response variable Y and a set of p predictors, $x_1, \ldots, x_p$, based on observations $\{x_{i1}, \ldots, x_{ip}, Y_i\}_1^N$. We assume that the underlying data structure can be described by

$$Y = f(x_1, \ldots, x_p) + \varepsilon, \tag{9.1}$$

where f is an unknown smooth function and ε is the measurement error with mean zero but unknown distribution.

In ordinary linear regression, f is assumed to be of the form $f(x) = \sum_1^p x_i \beta_i$. Then, the estimation of the function f becomes a problem of estimating parameters β. Thanks to its simplicity, linear regression is among the most frequently used statistical techniques. In applications, however, the underlying data structure cannot always be summarized by a simple model, and hence the restrictive assumptions behind the simplicity may result in poor fits. Accordingly, alternatives to linear regression are of considerable interest for understanding the relationship between the covariates and the response. Nonparametric procedures using splines offer one solution to this problem. They are based on the idea that a smooth function can be well approximated by piecewise polynomials (see, e.g., De Boor, 1978). Here, we focus on two classes of models that are built upon the recursive partitioning technique. One is regression trees, and the other is multivariate adaptive regression splines (MARS, Friedman, 1991).

Regression trees fit a constant to the response within every terminal node, whereas adaptive splines use piecewise linear functions as the basis functions. The key difference between MARS and CART lies in the fact

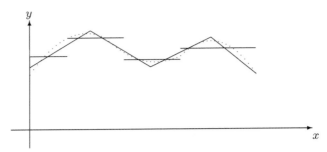

FIGURE 9.1. One-dimensional MARS (the thinner piecewise line) and CART (the step function) models. The dotted curve is the underlying smooth function.

that the regression function is continuous in MARS with respect to a continuous covariate, but not in CART. Therefore, MARS models are more appealing when continuity is a concern. In some applications such as image compression (e.g., Gersho and Gray, 1992, and Poggi and Olshen, 1995), extracting homogeneous predictive regions of the data is of scientific interest; hence regression trees are appropriate. Figure 9.1 offers a schematic comparison between MARS and CART models. An earlier version of MARS for one-dimensional smoothing was established by Friedman and Silverman (1989). The presentation here includes the modifications to MARS proposed by Zhang (1994).

9.1 Tree Representation of Spline Model and Analysis of Birth Weight

Before presenting the methods, let us see what results from the use of MARS for analyzing the Yale Pregnancy Outcome Study, as introduced in Chapter 2. In Section 3.2 we realized that two variables, x_7 (marijuana use) and x_8 (passive exposure to marijuana), have a substantial number of missing values. They were removed from the final logistic regression analysis at that time, and now we again do not consider them. Hence, the present analysis includes 13 of the 15 predictors in Table 2.1. The response is birth weight in grams. As in the previous logistic regression, we use 3,836 complete observations out of the entire 3,861 subjects.

9.1 Tree Representation of Spline Model and Analysis of Birth Weight

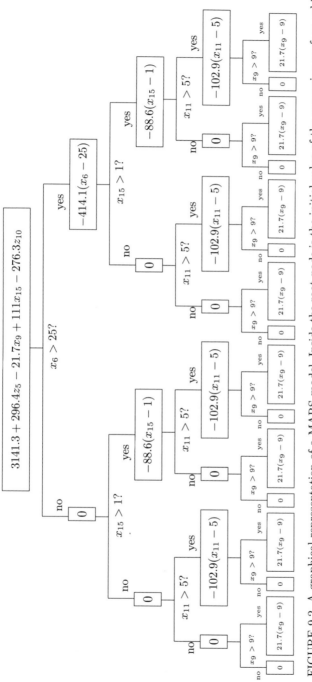

FIGURE 9.2. A graphical representation of a MARS model. Inside the root node is the initial value of the regression surface, which is recursively added by the values inside the offspring nodes.

Figure 9.2 presents a fitted regression model using MARS for our data, where z_5 and z_{10} are dummy variables defined in Section 3.2, indicating a White woman and the DES use of the pregnant woman's mother, respectively. An explicit mathematical formula for the MARS model will be given in (9.41). The representation of the MARS model in Figure 9.2 shows the relationship between adaptive splines and classification trees, because they both are based on the recursive partitioning of the domain formed by the covariates.

At the top of Figure 9.2, which we used to call the root node, is the function

$$3141.3 + 296.4z_5 - 21.7x_9 + 111x_{15} - 276.3z_{10}. \qquad (9.2)$$

It can be used to calculate the initial value of predicting the birth weight for any newborn. For instance, if the mother is a White nonsmoking woman ($z_5 = 1, x_9 = 0$), her mother did not use DES ($z_{10} = 0$), and she was pregnant once before ($x_{15} = 1$), then her newborn is assigned an initial weight of $3141.3+296.4*1-21.7*0+111*1-276.3*0 = 3548.7$ grams. At the second layer, there is a zero inside the left daughter node and $-414.1(x_6 - 25)$ inside the right daughter node, as separated by the question of "$x_6 > 25$?" This means, for example, that $-414.1 * (27 - 25) = -828.2$ grams will be reduced from the newborn's initially assigned weight if his or her mother had 27 years of education. However, no change is made if the mother had no more than 25 years of education. Other nodes in Figure 9.2 can be interpreted similarly.

In summary, on average, White babies are 296.4 grams heavier than the others, and the DES use of the pregnant woman's mother reduces a newborn's weight by 276.3 grams. We see negative effects of high levels of education (more than 25 years, $x_6 > 25$), parity ($x_{15} > 1$), and gravidity ($x_{11} > 5$). Two terms involve x_9, the number of cigarettes smoked. One ($-21.7x_9$) appears in the root node, and the other $[21.7(x_9 - 9)]$ in the terminal nodes. The sum of these two terms suggests that the number of cigarettes smoked has a negative effect when the number is beyond a half pack of cigarettes per day.

The tree representation in Figure 9.2 is left and right balanced because we have an additive spline model. That is, each term involves only one predictor. However, in the presence of product terms of two or more predictors, the tree representation of a MARS model is not necessarily balanced, which is similar to those classification trees that we have seen before.

9.2 Regression Trees

In Chapter 4 we have pointed out that we need a within-node impurity or, directly, a node splitting criterion to grow a large tree and then a cost-complexity criterion to prune a large tree. These general guidelines apply whenever we attempt to develop tree-based methods.

For a continuous response, a natural choice of node impurity for node τ is the within-node variance of the response:

$$i(\tau) = \sum_{\text{subject } i \in \tau} (Y_i - \bar{Y}(\tau))^2, \qquad (9.3)$$

where $\bar{Y}$ is the average of Y_i's within node τ. To split a node τ into its two daughter nodes, τ_L and τ_R, we maximize the split function

$$\phi(s, \tau) = i(\tau) - i(\tau_L) - i(\tau_R), \qquad (9.4)$$

where s is an allowable split. Unlike the goodness of split in (2.3), the split function in (9.4) does not need weights. Furthermore, we can make use of $i(\tau)$ to define the tree cost as

$$R(\mathcal{T}) = \sum_{\tau \in \tilde{\mathcal{T}}} i(\tau) \qquad (9.5)$$

and then substitute it into (4.7) to form the cost-complexity.

To compare with the use of MARS, we construct regression trees for the birth weight data analyzed in the preceding section. Figure 9.3 outlines the profile of this large tree.

Figure 9.4 displays the result of pruning the tree in Figure 9.3. It plots the tree size (the bottom x-axis) and the complexity parameter (the top x-axis) against the deviance (the y-axis), or equivalently, the variance.

We can see that there is a relatively large drop of deviance at the complexity parameter 2.5E6, and the decrement is gradual after that point. Pruning the tree with the complexity parameter 2.5E6 leads to the final tree in Figure 9.5, which also depicts the empirical distributions of birth weight within all terminal nodes. In this final tree, the number of cigarettes smoked per day is used twice, once at 8 and the other time at 1. One may change these cutoff values to 9 and 0, respectively, to simplify the interpretation, which would correspond to smoking half a pack and to not smoking.

Both MARS and CART confirm that White women tend to deliver heavier infants. Women smoking about or more than half a pack of cigarettes per day give birth to smaller infants. The tree in Figure 9.5 indicates that women having delivered before subsequently deliver larger infants. In the MARS model, the number of previous pregnancies contributes to the infant birth weight as follows:

$$\begin{cases} 0 & \text{if no previous pregnancy,} \\ 111 & \text{if one previous pregnancy,} \\ 25 & \text{if two previous pregnancies,} \\ -66 & \text{if three previous pregnancies,} \end{cases}$$

110   9. Regression Trees and Adaptive Splines for a Continuous Response

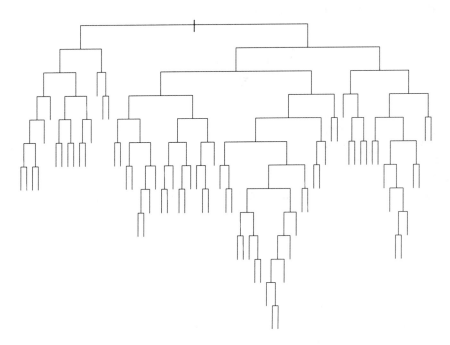

FIGURE 9.3. The profile of an initial regression tree for birth weight

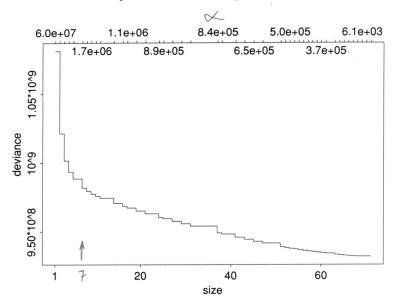

FIGURE 9.4. Subtree complexity and deviance

9.2 Regression Trees   111

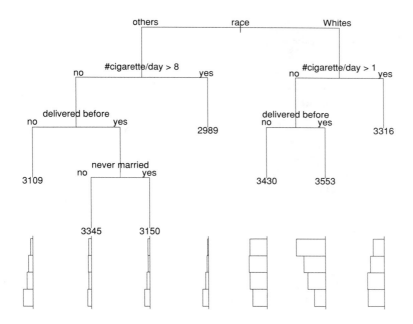

FIGURE 9.5. A pruned regression tree for birth weight. On the top is the tree structure with the average birth weights displayed for the terminal nodes and at the bottom the within-terminal-node histograms of birth weight.

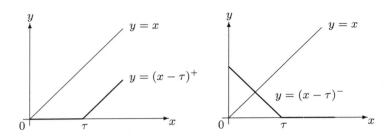

FIGURE 9.6. Truncated basis functions

providing a more specific relationship between the history of pregnancy and birth weight.

The computation here is done in SPLUS. A sample code of our computation is given below. The response variable is labeled as btw and all predictors as allpreds. To reduce the computation burden, we grow the initial tree, requiring the minimal node size to be 80.

```
birth.tree <- tree(btw ~ allpreds, minsize=80, mincut=40)
plot(birth.tree, type="u")
plot(prune.tree(birth.tree))
final.tree <- prune.tree(birth.tree, k=2500000)
tree.screens()
plot(final.tree, type="u")
text(final.tree)
tile.tree(final.tree)
```

9.3 The Profile of MARS Models

Building a MARS model is a complicated process, and hence it is very helpful to know what kinds of models MARS produces. For readers who are interested mainly in the applications, this section should provide enough background for their needs.

MARS models can be reorganized to have the form of

$$\beta_0 + \sum \beta_{ij}(x_i - \tau_j)^* + \sum_{i \neq k} \beta_{ijkl}(x_i - \tau_j)^*(x_k - \tau_l)^* + \cdots, \quad (9.6)$$

where $(x_i - \tau_j)^*$ is either the negatively truncated function $(x_i - \tau_j)^+$ or the positively truncated one $(x_i - \tau_j)^-$. Here, for any number a, let $a^+ = \max(0, a)$ and $a^- = a^+ - a$. Figure 9.6 displays these two truncated functions.

Note that the sum of multiplicative terms in model (9.6) is over different predictors, as is dictated by the conditions such as $i \neq k$ for the second-

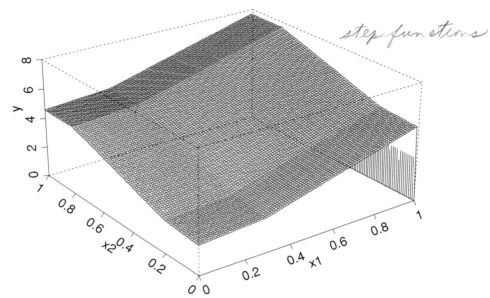

FIGURE 9.7. MARS model: $2.5 + 4(x_1 - 0.3)^+ - (x_1 - 0.3)^- + 4(x_2 - 0.2)^+ - (x_2 - 0.2)^- - 4(x_2 - 0.8)^+$.

order terms. In other words, the same predictor is not allowed to appear more than once in a single term. As a consequence, in the one-dimensional case, model (9.6) becomes

$$\beta_0 + \sum_{k=1}^{M} \beta_k (x - \tau_k)^*, \tag{9.7}$$

because we cannot have higher-order multiplicative terms without using the same predictor more than once. Model (9.7) is a sum of truncated line segments and is called a piecewise linear function, as illustrated by Figure 9.1. It is noteworthy that model (9.7) would be equivalent to a regression tree model if the truncated function $(x - \tau_k)^*$ were replaced with an indicator function $I(x > \tau_k)$ defined in (6.1) in Section 6.1. A linear combination of indicator functions produces a step function, as is also depicted in Figure 9.1.

Furthermore, model (9.6) can be regarded as a generalization of regression trees. The two types of model are identical if the predictors are categorical. When the predictors are continuous, model (9.6) can be converted into a regression tree model by changing the truncated linear functions into the indicator functions.

With two continuous predictors, x_1 and x_2, Figures 9.7 and 9.8 display two representative MARS models. What we should notice from Figures 9.7 and 9.8 is that the predictor space of (x_1, x_2) is partitioned into several

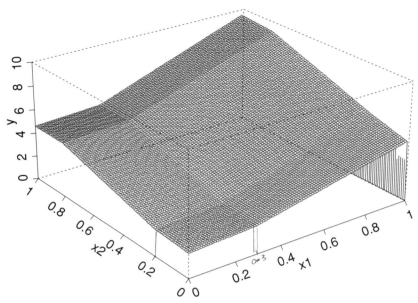

FIGURE 9.8. MARS model: $2.5 + 5(x_1 - 0.3)^+ - (x_1 - 0.3)^- + 4(x_2 - 0.2)^+ - (x_2 - 0.2)^- - 4(x_2 - 0.8)^+ + 2(x_1 - 0.3)^+(x_2 - 0.2)^+ - 5(x_1 - 0.3)^+(x_2 - 0.2)^-$.

rectangles. In regression trees, a flat plane is used to fit the data within each rectangle, and obviously the entire fit is not continuous in the borders of the rectangles. In contrast, the MARS model is continuous, and within each rectangle, it may or may not be a simple plane. For instance, the MARS model in Figure 9.7 consists of six connected planes. However, the MARS model in Figure 9.8 has both simple planes and "twisted" surfaces with three pieces of each. The twisted surfaces result from the last two second-order terms, and they are within the rectangles (i) $x_1 > 0.3$ and $x_2 < 0.2$, (ii) $x_1 > 0.3$ and $0.2 < x_2 < 0.8$, and (iii) $x_1 > 0.3$ and $x_2 > 0.8$. Figure 9.9 provides a focused view of the typical shape of a twisted surface.

What are the differences between the MARS model (9.6) and the ordinary linear regression model? In the ordinary linear model, we decide a priori how many and what terms are to be entered into the model. However, we do not know how many terms to include in a MARS model prior to the data modeling. In Figure 9.1, the MARS model is represented by four line segments, but it could be three, five, or any number of segments. In practice, we do assign a limit, such as 20 or 50, to the maximum number of terms that can be included in a MARS model, depending on the data dimension. The choice of this limit is much easier to choose than is specifying the exact number of terms in a model, and its impact is relatively small in the model selection. Another key difference resides in that every term in a linear model is fully determined, while it is partially specified in

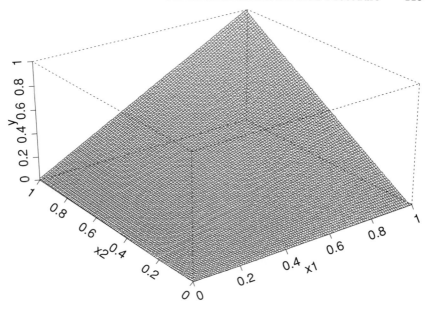

FIGURE 9.9. A twisted surface: $x_1 x_2$.

the MARS model. Particularly, the location of the knot, τ_k, in $(x - \tau_k)^*$ needs to be determined from the data. This is why (9.6) is an adaptive spline model. Furthermore, the predictors x_i need to be selected during the course of building model (9.6), and whether multiplicative terms, such as $(x_1 - \tau_1)^+(x_2 - \tau_2)^+$, prove to be necessary is also data driven. In ordinary linear regression, however, these decisions are to be made before the model estimation. The common feature shared by (9.6) and the ordinary linear regression model is that the coefficient β's will be linear coefficients after the other model parameters are fixed.

9.4 Modified MARS Forward Procedure

MARS was originally developed by Friedman (1991). In this section we present a modified MARS forward algorithm described by Zhang (1994). The two chief differences between the original and the modified versions are the exact solution to the best knot and the constraints between knot locations. During this forward process, we need to understand two issues: how to enter predictors into the MARS model and how to find the best knots.

First, we present the outline of the algorithm in order to quickly grasp the process by which the terms are added into the model (9.6). Then, we elaborate all steps.

116   9. Regression Trees and Adaptive Splines for a Continuous Response

The Forward Algorithm

0. Enter the intercept term, β_0. Namely, include a constant, 1, as the first basis function.

1. Find the combination of predictor x_i and knot τ_1 that gives the best fit to the data when the pair of basis functions

$$(x_i - \tau_1)^+ \text{ and } (x_i - \tau_1)^-$$

is added to the model.

2. If K basis functions have been entered, find the combination of predictor x_k, knot τ_l, and an existing term, denoted by s, that yields the best fit to the data when

$$s(x_k - \tau_l)^+ \text{ and } s(x_k - \tau_l)^-$$

are added to the model.

3. Repeat step 2 until the maximum number of basis functions have been collected.

Step 0 is trivial, although we should note that the value of β_0 changes during the course of adding more terms. For the remaining three steps, we need to clarify the meaning of the best fit to the data:

Definition 9.1 *The Least Squares Criterion.*
For any regression function $f(\mathbf{x}; \theta)$ depending on the pair of predictors, $\mathbf{x}$, and a set of unknown parameters, θ, we search for a set of solutions, $\hat{\theta}$, that minimize the residual sum of squares (RSS)

$$\sum_{1}^{N}(Y_i - f(\mathbf{x}_i; \theta))^2 \qquad (9.8)$$

over the entire domain of θ. In other words, <u>our parameter estimates are based on the least squares criterion</u>.

To understand what is involved in step 1, it is helpful to know precisely what the MARS model looks like at this step. After step 0, the MARS model includes a constant term, and the best constant based on the least squares criterion (9.8) is $\bar{Y}$, the sample average of Y. In step 1, we consider adding a pair of

$$(x_i - \tau_1)^+ \text{ and } (x_i - \tau_1)^-$$

into the existing model that has the constant term only. Thus, the candidate MARS model in the present step is of the form

$$\beta_0 + \beta_1(x_i - \tau)^+ + \beta_2(x_i - \tau)^-, \qquad (9.9)$$

9.4 Modified MARS Forward Procedure

TABLE 9.1. Step-by-Step Cumulation of a MARS Model. The newly added terms are underlined.

Step	Fitted Model
0	-0.71
1	$0.68 \underline{-2.18x_2 - 7.1(x_2 - 0.72)^+}$
2(a)	$-0.41 - 2.18x_2 - 7.92(x_2 - 0.72)^+ \underline{+1.28x_1 + 3.59(x_1 - 0.55)^+}$
2(b)	$-0.4 - 3.37x_2 - 8.21(x_2 - 0.72)^+ + 1.36x_1 + 3.05(x_1 - 0.55)^+$ $\underline{+2.65x_2x_3 - 30.4x_2(x_3 - 0.94)^+}$
2(c)	$-0.39 - 3.17x_2 - 8.24(x_2 - 0.72)^+ + 1.32x_1 + 3.09(x_1 - 0.55)^+$ $+2.56x_2x_3 - 37x_2(x_3 - 0.94)^+ \underline{-0.4x_2x_4 - 0.81x_2(x_4 - 0.84)^+}$
⋮	⋮

for some $i = 1, \ldots, p$, and a knot τ. Note here that

$$(x_i - \tau)^- = (x_i - \tau)^+ - (x_i - \tau),$$

which implies that $(x_i - \tau)^-$ is a linear combination of $(x_i - \tau)$ and $(x_i - \tau)^+$. As a result, we do not need two truncated functions in (9.9). For computational consideration, it is easy to replace (9.9) with an equivalent model

$$\beta_0 + \beta_1 x_i + \beta_2 (x_i - \tau)^+. \tag{9.10}$$

Model (9.10) is preferred for two reasons. First, knot τ, a nonlinear parameter, appears only once, and this fact makes it easier to derive the best knot. Second, it is clear from (9.10) that we cannot always add a pair of basis functions, due to linear dependency. After x_i is entered into the model, we can add only a single term, $(x_i - \tau)^+$ (or alternatively $(x_i - \tau)^-$), as we consider additional basis functions generated by the sample predictor. However, for conceptual consistency we did not raise this issue in the description of step 2.

In Section 9.9 we will present a few numerical examples. For instance, in Example 9.4 we will use the MARS model to fit a three-dimensional model. Particularly, Table 9.1 offers a taste of how the MARS model is accumulated gradually for that example.

The most important technical question is, How do we find the best knot τ in conjunction with the predictor x_i? We defer the answer to Section 9.6. Instead, we address an easier question first, What happens after the best τ is found, together with its associate predictor? Model (9.10) is a linear model with respect to the coefficient β's. Because we use the least squares criterion, the estimation of β's is a standard process in fitting the linear models.

Step 2 is a further step to enlarging an existing MARS model. After a pair of basis functions, say x_1 and $(x_1 - \tau_1)^+$, are produced by step 1, there are three ways by which the existing model can be expanded. This is because the new pair can be associated with one of the three existing basis functions in (9.10). When the new pair of basis functions are multiplied by the constant basis function, they remain the same in the larger model. The resulting MARS model is one of

$$\beta_0 + \beta_1 x_1 + \beta_2 (x_1 - \tau_1)^+ + \beta_3 x_i + \beta_4 (x_i - \tau)^+, \text{ for } i \neq 1, \qquad (9.11)$$

and

$$\beta_0 + \beta_1 x_1 + \beta_2 (x_1 - \tau_1)^+ + \beta_3 (x_1 - \tau)^+. \qquad (9.12)$$

However, if the new pair of basis functions are multiplied by x_1, a pair of multiplicative basis functions (not the original basis functions) are attached to the existing model as follows:

$$\beta_0 + \beta_1 x_1 + \beta_2 (x_1 - \tau_1)^+ + \beta_3 x_1 x_i + \beta_4 x_1 (x_i - \tau)^+, \qquad (9.13)$$

where $i \neq 1$. Similarly, the new pair can be merged with $(x_1 - \tau_1)^+$, and this leads to the model

$$\beta_0 + \beta_1 x_1 + \beta_2 (x_1 - \tau_1)^+ + \beta_3 (x_1 - \tau_1)^+ x_i + \beta_4 (x_1 - \tau_1)^+ (x_i - \tau)^+, \qquad (9.14)$$

where $i \neq 1$. The best of models (9.11)–(9.14) is then selected in step 2. Step 3 repeats step 2 and keeps expanding the existing model by adding one or two new terms and leaving the existing terms intact. The new terms can be viewed as the product of a new pair of basis functions and one of the existing basis functions.

These forward steps can produce a large collection of basis functions. In practice, we stop the process when we are certain that the number of basis functions is well beyond a reasonable model size in accordance with the data. Furthermore, we also restrict the highest order of the multiplicative terms. In most applications, the third order appears to be reasonably high.

We then face the same issue as in the context of classification trees. What do we do about such a large MARS model? Obviously, we need to delete some of the basis functions. Fortunately, this backward elimination is easier than tree pruning, at least at a conceptual level. This is the topic of Section 9.5.

9.5 MARS Backward-Deletion Step

As in Section 9.4, we will first outline the backward algorithm, and then explain the steps in detail. The most important concept in this step is the generalized cross-validation criterion, as defined below.

The Backward Algorithm

0. Begin with the MARS model that contains all, say M, basis functions generated from the forward algorithm.

1. Delete the existing nonconstant basis function that makes the least contribution to the model according to the least squares criterion.

2. Repeat step 1 until only the constant basis remains in the model.

Suppose that we start with a 5-basis-function model

$$f_1(\mathbf{x}) = \beta_0 + \beta_1 x_1 + \beta_2 (x_1 - \tau_1)^+ + \beta_3 (x_1 - \tau_1)^+ x_2 + \beta_4 (x_1 - \tau_1)^+ (x_2 - \tau)^+ \tag{9.15}$$

in step 0. One of the following four nonconstant basis functions,

$$x_1, (x_1 - \tau_1)^+, (x_1 - \tau_1)^+ x_2, \text{ and } (x_1 - \tau_1)^+ (x_2 - \tau)^+,$$

can be removed in step 1. If we remove x_1, the new model is

$$\beta_0 + \beta_1 (x_1 - \tau_1)^+ + \beta_2 (x_1 - \tau_1)^+ x_2 + \beta_3 (x_1 - \tau_1)^+ (x_2 - \tau)^+. \tag{9.16}$$

Fitting model (9.16) to the data, we have an RSS, denoted by RSS_1, as defined in (9.8). Similarly, we can sequentially remove any of the other three basis functions and obtain the respective RSS from RSS_2 to RSS_4. If, say, RSS_3 is the largest RSS, the third basis function, $(x_1 - \tau_1)^+ x_2$, is removed first. Then, we repeat the same process, beginning with

$$f_2(\mathbf{x}) = \beta_0 + \beta_1 x_1 + \beta_2 (x_1 - \tau_1)^+ + \beta_3 (x_1 - \tau_1)^+ (x_2 - \tau)^+.$$

After a total of 4 steps, we should reach the constant basis in the model. During this process, we have a sequence of five nested models, $f_k, k = 1, \ldots, 5$, which includes both the initial 5-basis-function model and the constant-basis model. These five models are candidates for the final model. The remaining question is, Which one should we select? The answer would be obvious if we had a criterion by which to judge them. Friedman and Silverman (1989), Friedman (1991), and Zhang (1994) use a modified version of the generalized cross-validation criterion originally proposed by Craven and Wahba (1979):

$$GCV(k) = \frac{\sum_{i=1}^{N} (Y_i - \hat{f}_k(\mathbf{x}_i))^2}{N[1 - (C(k)/N)]^2}, \tag{9.17}$$

where $\hat{f}_k$ comes from f_k by plugging in the fitted parameters, $k = 1, \ldots, 5$, and $C(k)$ reflects the model complexity as shall be specified below. The numerator of $GCV(k)$ is the RSS of model f_k, and hence $GCV(k)$ reflects both the lack of fit and the model complexity. Therefore, $GCV(k)$ is parallel to the cost-complexity in the tree-based methods. We use $GCV(k)$ as the optimal criterion for model selection, and the final MARS model should lead to the smallest GCV.

Based on the discussion in Friedman and Silverman (1989) and Friedman (1991), an empirically best choice for $C(k)$ is 3 to 5 times the number of the nonconstant basis functions in the corresponding model.

Model selection criteria are ways to balance the lack of fit, size of the model, and scientific interpretability. Why is this balance important? Two issues are noteworthy. One is bias (as opposed to precision), and the other is variance (as opposed to stability). A large model that is "wisely" chosen tends to have a smaller bias in predicting the outcome, but it also suffers a greater variability. The backward-deletion procedure is designed to find the optimal compromise between these two factors.

So far, we have presented only a "big picture" of the MARS algorithm. In the subsequent sections, we will discuss in detail some technical issues that we must deal with when developing this methodology.

9.6 The Best Knot*

At the technical level, the most difficult part of the MARS algorithm is to locate the best knot in steps 1 and 2 of the forward algorithm, which is where we spend most of the computation time. The understanding of this section requires familiarity with linear algebra and linear regression.

The linearly truncated functions displayed in Figure 9.6 are the simplest nonlinear functions, but we still need to pay special attention to the knot that is a nonlinear parameter. Particularly, the truncated functions are not differentiable at the knot. Hence, a general optimization routine is not applicable for locating knots. Here, we derive an explicit formula for the best knot based on the ideas of Hinkley (1971), Friedman and Silverman (1989), and Zhang (1991). Our line of derivation is adopted from Zhang (1994).

Note that step 1 of the forward algorithm stated in Section 9.4 is a special case of the second step. We need to introduce vector and matrix notations and clearly formulate the problem involved in step 2.

When entering step 2, we assume that we have found K basis functions. Applying each of the K basis functions to the N observations, we obtain K corresponding basis vectors, denoted by $\mathbf{b}_0, \ldots, \mathbf{b}_{K-1}$. For instance, the first basis function is the constant 1. Thus, the first basis vector, $\mathbf{b}_0$, is an N-vector of all ones. Moreover, if $(x_i - \tau_1)^+$ is the second basis function, then
$$\mathbf{b}_1 = ((x_{1i} - \tau_1)^+, \ldots, (x_{Ni} - \tau_1)^+)'.$$
For convenience, we also write the vector above as
$$(\mathbf{x}^{(i)} - \tau_1 \mathbf{1})^+,$$

where $\mathbf{x}^{(i)} = (x_{1i}, \ldots, x_{Ni})'$ and $\mathbf{1} = \mathbf{b}_0 = (1, \ldots, 1)'$.

Now, we need to find another pair of basis functions that gives the best fit to the data when the basis functions are merged with one of the existing basis functions. Under the new notation, this means the following. Suppose that the basis functions under consideration are x_k and $(x_k - \tau)^+$ (note their equivalence to $(x_k - \tau)^+$ and $(x_k - \tau)^-$). They generate two basis vectors, $\mathbf{x}^{(k)}$ and $(\mathbf{x}^{(k)} - \tau\mathbf{1})^+$. After merging these two basis vectors with one of the existing basis vectors, we consider adding the following two basis vectors,

$$\mathbf{b}_l \circ \mathbf{x}^{(k)} \text{ and } \mathbf{b}_l \circ (\mathbf{x}^{(k)} - \tau\mathbf{1})^+, \tag{9.18}$$

$l = 0, \ldots, K$, into the existing model, where $\circ$ is the operation of multiplying two vectors componentwise. The pair (9.18) is ruled out automatically if $\mathbf{b}_l$ has $\mathbf{x}^{(k)}$ as a component. In addition, $\mathbf{b}_l \circ \mathbf{x}^{(k)}$ will be excluded if this vector is already in the model. To avoid these details, we assume that both basis vectors in (9.18) are eligible for inclusion. Let

$$B = (\mathbf{b}_0, \ldots, \mathbf{b}_K, \mathbf{b}_l \circ \mathbf{x}^{(k)}),$$
$$\mathbf{b}_{K+1}(\tau) = \mathbf{b}_l \circ (\mathbf{x}^{(k)} - \tau\mathbf{1})^+,$$

and

$$\mathbf{r} = (I - PP')\mathbf{Y},$$

where $\mathbf{Y} = (Y_1, \ldots, Y_N)'$, $PP' = B(B'B)^{-1}B'$, and $P'P$ is an identity matrix. Thus, $\mathbf{r}$ is the residual vector when the existing K basis vectors and one new (fixed) basis vector are entered. For any given τ, if we also enter $\mathbf{b}_{K+1}(\tau)$ into the model, the least squares criterion equals

$$\|\mathbf{r}\|^2 - \frac{(\mathbf{r}'\mathbf{b}_{K+1}(\tau))^2}{\mathbf{b}'_{K+1}(\tau)(I - PP')\mathbf{b}_{K+1}(\tau)}. \tag{9.19}$$

The second term in (9.19) is a function of τ; but the first one is not and hence is irrelevant to the search for the best knot. Here comes the key task: We must find the best τ such that

$$h(\tau) = \frac{(\mathbf{r}'\mathbf{b}_{K+1}(\tau))^2}{\mathbf{b}'_{K+1}(\tau)(I - PP')\mathbf{b}_{K+1}(\tau)} \tag{9.20}$$

is maximized. Consequently, the residual sum of squares in (9.19) would be minimized.

The critical part is that we can express $h(\tau)$ in (9.20) as a more explicit function of τ if we restrict τ to an interval between two adjacent observed values of x_k. Without loss of generality, suppose that $x_{1k}, \ldots, x_{Nk}$ are in increasing order and that they are distinct. For $\tau \in [x_{jk}, x_{j+1,k})$, we have

$$\mathbf{b}_{K+1}(\tau) = (\mathbf{b}_l \circ \mathbf{x}_k)_{(-j)} - \tau \mathbf{b}_{l(-j)}, \tag{9.21}$$

where $\mathbf{v}_{(-j)} = (0, \ldots, 0, v_{j+1}, \ldots, v_N)'$ for any vector $\mathbf{v}$. Then, the numerator of $h(\tau)$ equals the square of

$$\mathbf{r}'(\mathbf{b}_l \circ \mathbf{x}_k)_{(-j)} - \tau \mathbf{r}' \mathbf{b}_{l(-j)}, \tag{9.22}$$

which is a linear function of τ because neither $\mathbf{r}'(\mathbf{b}_l \circ \mathbf{x}_k)_{(-j)}$ nor $\mathbf{r}' \mathbf{b}_{l(-j)}$ depends on τ. Furthermore, the denominator of $h(\tau)$ is

$$||(\mathbf{b}_l \circ \mathbf{x}_k)_{(-j)}||^2 - ||P'(\mathbf{b}_l \circ \mathbf{x}_k)_{(-j)}||^2 + \tau^2(||\mathbf{b}_{l(-j)}||^2 - ||P'\mathbf{b}_{l(-j)}||^2)$$
$$-2\tau(\mathbf{b}'_{l(-j)}(\mathbf{b}_l \circ \mathbf{x}_k)_{(-j)} - (\mathbf{b}_l \circ \mathbf{x}_k)'_{(-j)} PP' \mathbf{b}_{l(-j)}). \tag{9.23}$$

Thus, $h(\tau)$ is a ratio of two quadratic polynomials in τ specified in (9.22) and (9.23). Precisely,

$$h(\tau) = \frac{(c_{1j} - c_{2j}\tau)^2}{c_{3j} - 2c_{4j}\tau + c_{5j}\tau^2},$$

where

$$c_{1j} = \mathbf{r}'(\mathbf{b}_l \circ \mathbf{x}_k)_{(-j)}, \tag{9.24}$$
$$c_{2j} = \mathbf{r}' \mathbf{b}_{l(-j)}, \tag{9.25}$$
$$c_{3j} = ||(\mathbf{b}_l \circ \mathbf{x}_k)_{(-j)}||^2 - ||P'(\mathbf{b}_l \circ \mathbf{x}_k)_{(-j)}||^2, \tag{9.26}$$
$$c_{4j} = \mathbf{b}'_{l(-j)}(\mathbf{b}_l \circ \mathbf{x}_k)_{(-j)} - (\mathbf{b}_l \circ \mathbf{x}_k)'_{(-j)} PP' \mathbf{b}_{l(-j)}, \tag{9.27}$$
$$c_{5j} = ||\mathbf{b}_{l(-j)}||^2 - ||P'\mathbf{b}_{l(-j)}||^2. \tag{9.28}$$

The subscript j of these constants reminds us of the particular interval for τ. Some algebra reveals that the minimizer of $h(\tau)$ on the interval $[x_{jk}, x_{j+1,k}]$ is either x_{jk} or

$$\frac{c_{2j} c_{3j} - c_{1j} c_{4j}}{c_{2j} c_{4j} - c_{1j} c_{5j}}, \tag{9.29}$$

if the latter is indeed in the interval.

It is important to observe that finding the best knot is trivial if we have the constant c's ready. Fortunately, the calculation of these c's is not as complicated as it looks. Let us take c_{1j} and c_{4j} to illustrate what is involved in the process.

We start with $j = 1$ and calculate c_{11} and c_{41} by definition. Then, we move on to $j = 2$. It is easy to see that

$$c_{12} = c_{1j} - r_2 b_{2l} x_{2k}, \tag{9.30}$$

where $\mathbf{r} = (r_1, \ldots, r_N)'$ and $\mathbf{b}_l = (b_{1l}, \ldots, b_{Nl})'$. Similarly, for the first term of c_{42} we have

$$\mathbf{b}'_{l(-2)}(\mathbf{b}_l \circ \mathbf{x}_k)_{(-2)} = \mathbf{b}'_{l(-2)}(\mathbf{b}_l \circ \mathbf{x}_k)_{(-1)} - b_{2l}^2 x_{2k}.$$

For the second term of c_{4j}, we need to create two temporary $(K+1)$-vectors:

$$\mathbf{w}_{1j} = P'(\mathbf{b}_l \circ \mathbf{x}_k)_{(-j)},$$
$$\mathbf{w}_{2j} = P'\mathbf{b}_{l(-j)}.$$

Then

$$\mathbf{w}_{12} = \mathbf{w}_{11} - b_{2l}x_{2k}\mathbf{p}_{2\cdot},$$
$$\mathbf{w}_{22} = \mathbf{w}_{21} - b_{2l}\mathbf{p}_{2\cdot},$$

where $\mathbf{p}_{2\cdot}$ is the second row vector of P. Therefore,

$$c_{42} = c_{41} - b_{2l}^2 x_{2k} - b_{2l}\mathbf{w}'_{11}\mathbf{p}_{2\cdot} - b_{2l}x_{2k}\mathbf{w}'_{11}\mathbf{p}_{2\cdot} + b_{2l}^2 x_{2k}\|\mathbf{p}_{2\cdot}\|^2. \quad (9.31)$$

Why do we need the recurrent formulas (9.30) and (9.31)? If we obtained c_{11}, it takes two multiplications and one subtraction to derive c_{12}. Furthermore, if c_{41} is already prepared, it takes $5(K+1)$ steps to update the vectors $\mathbf{w}_{12}$ and $\mathbf{w}_{22}$; $3(K+1)$ operations for computing $\mathbf{w}'_{11}\mathbf{p}_{2\cdot}$, $x_{2k}\mathbf{w}'_{11}\mathbf{p}_{2\cdot}$, and $\|\mathbf{p}_{2\cdot}\|^2$; and hence $8(K+1) + 11$ operations altogether to reach c_{42}. The importance of this tedious counting lies in the fact that the number of operations needed to move from c_{11} to to c_{12} is a constant and that the number of operations from c_{41} to c_{42} is proportional to the number of existing basis functions. Moreover, the numbers of required operations are the same as we move from c_{1j} to $c_{1,j+1}$ and from c_{4j} to $c_{4,j+1}$. In fact, it takes fewer than $18K$ operations to update all c's from one interval to the next. Thus, the best knot associated with $\mathbf{x}_k$ and $\mathbf{b}_l$ can be found in a total of $18KN$ operations. There are at most Kp combinations of (k,l), implying that the best pair of basis functions can be found in about $18K^2pN$ steps. Therefore, if we plan to build a MARS model with no more than M terms, the total number of operations needed is on the order of M^3pN. This detail is relevant when we implement and further extend the algorithm.

We have explained in detail how to find the candidate knot within each interval of the observed data points. The general search strategy is to scan one interval at a time and keep the best knot.

9.7 Restrictions on the Knot*

9.7.1 Minimum Span

There is another technicality in implementing the MARS algorithm that we have not mentioned. In the previous section we attempted to find the best knot. In practice, especially when the signal-to-noise ratio is low, the MARS model could be vulnerable to the noise when the knots are too close to each other. To resolve this practical issue, Friedman and Silverman (1989,

Section 2.3) introduced a concept of minimum span by imposing a fixed number of observations between two adjacent eligible knots. The minimum span is m if at least m observations are required between the knots. Then, the next question is, How do we choose a reasonable minimum span? Based on a coin-tossing argument, Friedman and Silverman (1989) suggested

$$m = -\frac{1}{2.5} \log_2[-(1/N)\ln(1-\alpha)], \qquad (9.32)$$

where $0.01 \leq \alpha \leq 0.05$ in the one-dimensional case.

This is the idea: In the one-dimensional case, the underlying model is

$$Y_i = f(x_i) + \epsilon_i \quad (1 \leq i \leq N).$$

Although ϵ_i is as likely to be positive as negative, it has a good chance to hit a long run of either sign. Inside the region where a "long" run occurs, the spline would follow the run and deviate from the underlying function. Interestingly, the response of the spline to such a locally long run will not degrade the fit outside the problematic region if we place one knot at the beginning of the run, one at the end, and at least one in the middle (for possible curvature). If we expect the maximum length of the run in N binomial trials to be $L_{\max}$, we can avoid the problem by requiring a minimum span of $L_{\max}/3$ because we cannot place three knots within the run. To be a little bit conservative, we may take the minimum span as $L_{\max}/2.5$ instead. Unfortunately, we do not know $L_{\max}$. But with a certain degree of confidence we know how large it can get. Precisely, the probability of observing a run of length $L(\alpha) = -\log_2[-(1/N)\ln(1-\alpha)]$ or longer in N binomial trials is approximately α. Therefore, with the minimum span (9.32) the chance for the spline to experience difficulties is $\alpha\%$.

9.7.2 Maximal Correlation

Note, however, that the minimum span (9.32) is applicable when the data points are one unit apart. This is not the case in many, perhaps most, applications. With unequally spaced data points, it appears to be a good idea to impose a distance, not a number of observations, between eligible knots. Therefore, it should be adjusted by the factor $(x_N - x_1)/(N-1)$. Also, we may want to have an average of at least one observation that separates two adjacent knots. Based on these considerations, we should revise the minimum span in (9.32) as

$$m = \max\left\{-\frac{x_N - x_1}{2.5(N-1)} \log_2[-(1/N)\ln(1-\alpha)], \frac{1}{N}\sum_{i=1}^{3}(x_{N-i+1} - x_i)\right\}. \qquad (9.33)$$

The minimum span in (9.33) is a choice for the univariate splines; however, we are interested in multivariate splines. Zhang (1994) points out potential problems that may arise in the multivariate case. The design matrix involved in the MARS model degenerates as the number of terms in the model increases, and the problem becomes even more challenging as the knots get closer together. The use of minimum span cannot eliminate the degeneracy completely. Furthermore, in the multivariate case we must take into account relationships among the predictors, and some of the predictors may be categorical. The concept of minimum span needs to be redefined to consider what we would encounter in multivariate splines.

The following proposition of Zhang (1994) is an important clue for us to turn the concept of minimum span to a new one: maximal correlation.

Proposition 9.1 Suppose that x_i is an ordered predictor. For $x_{1i} \leq \tau \leq x_{Ni}$, let $\mathbf{b}(\tau) = (\mathbf{x}_i - \tau \mathbf{1})^+$. For $\tau_1 < \tau_2$, the correlation, $\rho(\tau_1, \tau_2)$, between $\mathbf{b}(\tau_1)$ and $\mathbf{b}(\tau_2)$ decreases as $\delta = \tau_2 - \tau_1$ increases.

Proof. It suffices to show that the derivative of ρ with respect to δ is nonnegative for any given τ_1.

Suppose that $x_j \leq \tau_1 < x_{j+1}$ and $x_k \leq \tau_1 + \delta < x_{k+1}$, for some $1 \leq j \leq k < N$. Let $Y_i = x_i - \tau_1$, $i = 1, \ldots, N$. Then, $\rho(\tau_1, \tau_1 + \delta)$ equals

$$\frac{\sum_{i>k} Y_i(Y_i - \delta) - \sum_{i>j} Y_i \sum_{i>k}(Y_i - \delta)/N}{([\sum_{i>j} Y_i^2 - (\sum_{i>j} Y_i)^2/N]\{\sum_{i>k}(Y_i - \delta)^2 - [\sum_{i>k}(Y_i - \delta)]^2/N\})^{1/2}}.$$

The derivative of $\rho(\tau_1, \tau_1 + \delta)$ with respect to δ has the same sign as

$$\left[-\sum_{i>k} Y_i + (1 - k/N) \sum_{i>j} Y_i\right] \left\{\sum_{i>k}(Y_i - \delta)^2 - \left[\sum_{i>k}(Y_i - \delta)\right]^2/N\right\}$$

$$+ (k/N) \sum_{i>k}(Y_i - \delta) \left[\sum_{i>k} Y_i(Y_i - \delta) - \sum_{i>j} Y_i \sum_{i>k}(Y_i - \delta)/N\right]. \quad (9.34)$$

After some manipulations, it is easy to see that the expression (9.34) equals

$$\frac{1}{N} \left\{\sum_{i>k}(Y_i - \delta)^2 - \left[\sum_{i>k}(Y_i - \delta)\right]^2/(N - k)\right\} \left(\sum_{i=j+1}^{k} Y_i - k\delta\right),$$

which does not exceed zero, because $\delta \geq Y_i$ for $i \leq k$.

Geometrically, the proposition can be viewed as follows. Suppose that x_i takes an integer value from 1 to 5 and $\tau_1 = 1$. We can make a scatter plot of 5 points using $\mathbf{b}(1)$ as the abscissa and $\mathbf{b}(\tau)$ as the ordinate. See Figure 9.10. As τ moves farther away from 1, the resulting 5 points become more and more near a flat line, indicating that the correlation between $\mathbf{b}(\tau)$ and $\mathbf{b}(1)$ decreases as τ increases.

The proposition above reveals that the closer together the knots are, the more correlated are the terms added to the model. In other words, imposing

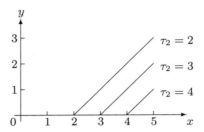

FIGURE 9.10. Correlation between basis vectors

a minimum span is one way to control the correlation among adopted bases. Hence, it would be more direct to control the correlation in the first place.

It is noteworthy to point out that the proposition does not imply that $\rho(\tau_1, \tau_1 + \delta_1) > \rho(\tau_2, \tau_2 + \delta_2)$ for $\delta_1 < \delta_2$ when $\tau_1 \neq \tau_2$. Thus, we need to watch out for the potential boundary effects of the correlation $\rho(\tau_1, \tau_2)$. To illustrate the situation in the univariate model, suppose that the model has two knots τ_1 and τ_2 ($\tau_1 > \tau_2$), with τ_1 in the interior and τ_2 near the boundary; we consider the inclusion of a third knot τ_3. The candidate τ_3 can be chosen closer to τ_2 than to τ_1 without violating the correlation threshold, because $\rho(\tau_2, \tau_2 + \delta)$ tends to be less than $\rho(\tau_1, \tau_1 + \delta)$. By fixing δ and varying τ, it can be seen graphically that $\rho(\tau, \tau + \delta)$ increases as τ moves from the left to the right. As a consequence, knots on the left edge of the interval are presumably allowed to be closer together.

To resolve this potential problem, Zhang (1994) introduced a modified correlation. Suppose $\tau_1, \ldots, \tau_k$ are the knots that have already been included in the model, and the next knot τ, associated with a predictor x_i, is to be determined. Let ρ_+ be the generalized linear correlation between $(\mathbf{x}_i - \tau\mathbf{1})^+$ and the previously adopted bases and let ρ_- be similarly defined using $(\mathbf{x}_i - \tau\mathbf{1})^-$. Precisely,

$$\rho_-(\tau) = 1 - \frac{\|(I - PP')\mathbf{b}_-(\tau)\|^2}{\|\mathbf{b}_-(\tau) - \bar{\mathbf{b}}_-(\tau)\mathbf{1}\|^2}, \quad (9.35)$$

$$\rho_+(\tau) = 1 - \frac{\|(I - PP')\mathbf{b}(\tau)\|^2}{\|\mathbf{b}(\tau) - \bar{\mathbf{b}}(\tau)\mathbf{1}\|^2}, \quad (9.36)$$

where a bar denotes the average of a vector, and $\mathbf{b}_-(\tau) = (\mathbf{x}_i - \tau\mathbf{1})^-$.

The modified correlation is defined by $\max(\rho_+, \rho_-)$. We have observed that ρ_+ tends to be larger when τ is near the right end, while ρ_- tends to be larger at the left end. As a result, the use of $\max(\rho_+, \rho_-)$ discourages knots near either end. In what follows, ρ will be referred to as the modified correlation.

9.7.3 Patches to the MARS Forward Algorithm

Here, we incorporate the maximal correlation into the MARS forward algorithm.

In step 0, we initialize an outset maximal correlation, R^*. For most users, $R^* = 0.9999$ should be a fine choice. This R^* safeguards us from a numerical correlation too close to (perhaps even greater than) 1.

In step 1, after the first knot τ_1 associated with a predictor x_{i_1} is found, we define the onset maximal correlation R through the minimum span L, associated with x_{i_1}, as follows:

$$R = \begin{cases} \max\{\rho(\tau_1 - L), \rho(\tau_1 + L)\}, & \text{if } x_{i_1 N} - L \geq \tau_1 \geq x_{i_1 1} + L, \\ \rho(\tau_1 - L), & \text{if } \tau_1 + L > x_{i_1 N}, \\ \rho(\tau_1 + L), & \text{otherwise,} \end{cases}$$

where $\rho(\tau)$ is the modified correlation coefficient induced by t and the knot τ_1. If $R > R^*$, set $R = R^*$; that is, R^* prevents R from being numerically almost 1.0.

When we add a new knot τ_k associated with a predictor x_{i_k} to the set of knots $\tau_1, \ldots, \tau_{k-1}$ in step 2, the modified correlation coefficient $\rho(\tau_k)$, induced by τ_k and the knots $\tau_1, \ldots, \tau_{k-1}$, must be less than the current R. As more knots are inserted into the model, the modified correlation induced by the new candidate knot and knots already in the model generally increases. Therefore, R should show an increase as needed, although it is never allowed to exceed R^*. A tentative scheme for making R increase is to calculate a temporary $\tilde{R}$ that is analogous to R in step 1:

$$\tilde{R} = \begin{cases} \max\{\rho(\tau_k - L), \rho(\tau_k + L)\}, & \text{if } x_{i_k N} - L > \tau_k > x_{i_k 1} + L, \\ \rho(\tau_k - L), & \text{if } \tau_k + L > x_{i_k N}, \\ \rho(\tau_k + L), & \text{otherwise.} \end{cases}$$

We then update R with $\tilde{R}$ if $\tilde{R}$ is indeed between R and R^*.

Updating R requires the calculation of ρ at different locations. Would this be a serious computational burden? No. It is obvious that the denominators and the numerators of $\rho_-(\tau)$ and $\rho_+(\tau)$ can be updated in a manner analogous to the approach used for (9.23)–(9.31). As a result, we are able to check the acceptability of an optimal knot at the same time we are locating it.

9.8 Smoothing Adaptive Splines*

We assume in model (9.1) that the underlying function f is smooth. On the contrary, the truncated spline basis functions are not smooth nor is the MARS model (9.6). Although this is not a major problem, it has apparently caused enough concern. Two types of solutions are available. One is to

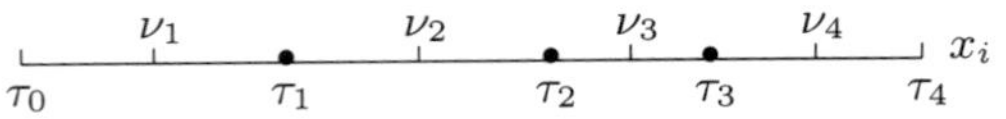

FIGURE 9.11. Placement of artificial knots

determine the model structure with the linearly truncated basis functions and then replace the basis functions with the smooth cubic functions, as shall be discussed in Section 9.8.1. The other approach is more dramatic and makes direct use of the cubic basis functions. This will be discussed in Section 9.8.2.

9.8.1 Smoothing the Linearly Truncated Basis Functions

Friedman (1991) described an ad hoc approach that repairs a MARS model. The repaired model has continuous derivatives. If we only need a model that is differentiable, we can use the approach taken by Tishler and Zang (1981) and Zhang (1991).

Suppose that x_i is involved in the model, and say, three distinct knots, $\tau_1 < \tau_2 < \tau_3$, are placed on x_i. Also, assume that the minimum and maximum of x_i are τ_0 and τ_4. Then, we insert an artificial knot in the middle of two adjacent τ's, namely,

$$\nu_i = (\tau_{j-1} + \tau_j)/2, \quad (j = 1, \ldots, 4).$$

The placement of ν is illustrated in Figure 9.11. Next, we replace the basis function $(x_i - \tau_j)^+$ $(j = 1, 2, 3)$ in the original MARS model with

$$\begin{cases} 0 & x_i \leq \nu_j, \\ \frac{2\nu_{j+1} + \nu_j - 3\nu_j}{(\nu_{j+1} - \nu_j)^2}(x_i - \nu_j)^2 + \frac{2\nu_j - \nu_{j+1} - \nu_j}{(\nu_{j+1} - \nu_j)^3}(x_i - \nu_j)^3 & \nu_j < x_i < \nu_{j+1}, \\ x_i - \nu_j & x_i \geq \nu_{j+1}. \end{cases}$$

After the replacement is done, we can reestimate the coefficients of the modified model from the data. Then the model has continuous derivatives.

9.8.2 Cubic Basis Functions

In Section 9.4 we have used x and $(x - \tau)^+$ as the seed basis functions. If instead, we built the spline model by attaching

$$\beta_1 x + \beta_2 x^2 + \beta_3 x^3 + \beta_4 [(x - \tau)^+]^3$$

to an existing basis function, we would end up with a cubic adaptive spline model. The function $[(x - \tau)^+]^3$ has a continuous derivative, and so does the resulting spline model. The key question is, Can we still find the best knot efficiently? The answer is yes if we restrict the candidate knots to the observed data points. There seems to be little benefit in removing this restriction for the cubic splines.

Following the discussion in Section 9.6, suppose that $\mathbf{b}_0, \ldots, \mathbf{b}_K$ are basis vectors already included in the model and that the new set of basis vectors,

$$\mathbf{x}_k, \mathbf{x}_k^2, \mathbf{x}_k^3, \text{ and } [(\mathbf{x}_k - \tau\mathbf{1})^+]^3,$$

is multiplied by a previous basis vector $\mathbf{b}_l$. Here, the power of a vector is with respect to the components of the vector.

Recall from (9.19) and (9.20) that the RSS due to the MARS model including both the existing and the new basis functions is $\|\mathbf{r}\|^2 - h(\tau)$, with $h(\tau)$ defined in (9.20). Here, $\mathbf{r}$ is the residual vector when $\mathbf{b}_0, \ldots, \mathbf{b}_K, \mathbf{x}_k$, $\mathbf{x}_k^2$, and $\mathbf{x}_k^3$ are entered into the model. Note, however, that with the use of cubic basis functions we need to change $\mathbf{b}_{K+1}(\tau)$ in (9.21) to

$$[(\mathbf{b}_l \circ \mathbf{x}_k)_{(-j)} - \tau \mathbf{b}_{l(-j)}]^3.$$

The critical fact to realize is that we deal with a similar set of constant c's as defined in (9.24)–(9.28) when searching for the best knot from one observed data point to the next. For example, we need to update

$$\mathbf{r}'(\mathbf{b}_l \circ \mathbf{b}_l \circ \mathbf{b}_l \circ \mathbf{x}_k \circ \mathbf{x}_k \circ \mathbf{x}_k)_{(-j)}.$$

This is obviously more complicated than c_{1j}, but the principle is the same.

9.9 Numerical Examples

In this section we take a few simulated examples to illustrate the use and the interpretation of the adaptive spline model. First, we examine what happens when the data are purely noise; namely, there does not exist a deterministic functional structure. Then, we study three examples representing one-, two-, and three-dimensional functions. At the end, we revisit the model displayed in Figure 9.2 and explain how it was formulated.

Example 9.1 *Pure Noise.*

Before we use the MARS algorithm to build a model, it is important to probe whether the algorithm picks up false signals when none exists. The pure noise model is ideal for such an exercise. Friedman and Silverman (1989), Friedman (1991), and Zhang (1994), among others, have conducted many experiments and concluded that the MARS algorithm and its variants are very reliable for not falsely reporting signals. This assertion will be confirmed in example 9.4, where the final MARS model excludes all nuisance predictors that play no role in the underlying model.

Example 9.2 *Motorcycle Impact Data.*

This is a one-dimensional model with a challenging structure. Both Friedman and Silverman (1989) and Zhang (1994) used this example to illustrate the use of adaptive spline models. The name of the example reflects the fact that the data mimic those in a simulated experiment to investigate the efficacy of helmet use in motorcycle crashes (Silverman, 1985).

Suppose that the underlying function is of the form

$$f(x) = \begin{cases} 0 & \text{if } -0.2 \leq x < 0, \\ \sin[2\pi(1-x)^2] & \text{if } 0 \leq x \leq 1. \end{cases}$$

First, we take 50 random points from the interval $[-0.2, 1.0]$ and denote them by x_i, $i = 1, \ldots, 50$. Then, we generate a series of 50 random numbers from the normal distribution, namely, $\varepsilon_i \sim N[0, \max^2(0.05, x_i)]$, $i = 1, \ldots, 50$. Finally, the observation is the convolution of the signal, $f(x)$, and the noise, ε. That is,

$$Y_i = f(x_i) + \varepsilon_i, \quad i = 1, \ldots, 50.$$

It is interesting to note here that the noise variance is proportional to the magnitude of the predictor. Thus, this example attests to the use of adaptive spline models when the measurement errors are heterogeneous.

Figure 9.12 shows a plot of the simulated data (the dots) and the underlying function (the solid curve). Eight knots corresponding to 8 basis functions were added into the MARS model during the forward step in the order 0.12, 0.480, 0.817, −0.00656, 0.547, 0.345, 0.233, and 0.741. Four basis functions were removed on the basis of generalized cross-validation in the backward step. The selected MARS model is

$$0.0033 + 0.1832x - 9.0403(x + 0.00656)^+ + 14.6662(x - 0.12)^+ \\ - 10.9915(x - 0.547)^+ + 10.8185(x - 0.817)^+.$$

This fitted model is also plotted in Figure 9.12 (the dashed curve) along with a smoothed curve (the dotted one) resulting from the loess() function in SPLUS.

As shown by Figure 9.12, the MARS fit catches the shape of the underlying function quite well except for the artificial jump at the right end, which appears to be a result of three clustered, relatively large positive noises. The loess fit has problems at both ends, although the fit may be improved if we attempt to find the optimal bandwidth of this smoothing method. What is important to notice is that three of the four MARS knots are placed at the critical locations of the underlying function. The last knot appears to be the result of relatively high noise.

Figure 9.13 gives a detailed view of the residuals and the absolute errors. The residuals are the differences between the observation and the fit, whereas the absolute errors are the absolute differences between the true function value and the fitted value. Both panels of this figure suggest that the MARS model is preferable to the loess fit.

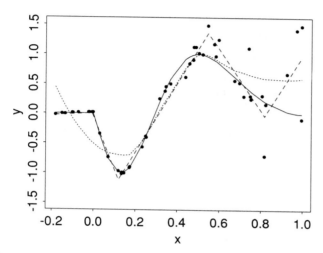

FIGURE 9.12. Motorcycle example: simulated data (the dots), the true function (the solid curve), the MARS fit (the dashed curve), and the loess fit (the dotted curve).

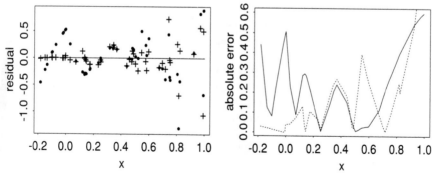

FIGURE 9.13. Residuals and absolute errors for the motorcycle data. The dots and the solid curve are from the loess fit. The plus signs and the dotted curves come from the MARS fit

For the present example, estimating the minimum and maximum of the underlying functions is the impetus to the original experiment (Silverman, 1985). Figure 9.12 shows that the MARS model gives a precise estimate of the minimum, while the `loess` offers a good estimate of the maximum. But both fits overestimate the other end of the function.

Example 9.3 *An Additive Model*

We use this example to illustrate an important point in building the MARS model: collinearity. Our data are simulated following the description of Hastie (1989) except that we used a higher noise level.

We simulated 100 observations from the model

$$Y_i = \frac{2}{3}\sin(1.3 x_{i1}) - \frac{9}{20} x_{i2}^2 + \varepsilon_i,$$

where x_{i1}, x_{i2}, and ε_i were generated from the standard normal distribution $N(0,1)$. The theoretical correlation between x_{i1} and x_{i2} is 0.4.

With two predictors, the MARS allows for the second-order product term. The selected MARS model is

$$0.77 - 6.14(x_1 - 0.48)^+ + 5.81(x_1 - 0.24) + 1.58 x_2 - 2.16(x_2 + 0.6)^+$$
$$-1.92(x_1 + 1.36)^+ (x_2 - 1.97)^+. \qquad (9.37)$$

Note that the original model is an additive model, but the MARS model includes an interaction term: $(x_1 + 1.36)^+ (x_2 - 1.97)^+$. This most likely is a result of the collinearity between x_1 and x_2, which confuses the MARS algorithm. How do we deal with this problem? First, let us forbid the use of the second-order product term. Then, a new MARS model is selected as follows:

$$0.45 - 1.73(x_1 - 0.48)^+ + 1.48(x_1 + 0.61)^+$$
$$+ 1.5 x_2 - 2.06(x_2 + 0.6)^+ - 2.21(x_2 - 1.49)^+. \qquad (9.38)$$

If we know the truth, model (9.38) is preferable to model (9.37). The question is, When do we forbid the use of higher-order product terms when the true model is not known? Friedman (1991) suggests comparing the GCV values obtained from various models for which different orders of interactions are considered. In this example, the GCV for model (9.37) is 1.37, whereas it is 1.28 for model (9.38). This indicates that the parsimonious model (9.38) serves us better.

In theory, the lower-order models constitute a subset of the class of high-order models. Due to the stepwise nature of the MARS algorithm, we do not necessarily end up with a better model by starting with a broader collection of models. In practice, we should build several MARS models by allowing different orders of interactions. Unless the GCV value suggests an improvement by a higher-order model, we always favor a lower-order one.

9.9 Numerical Examples

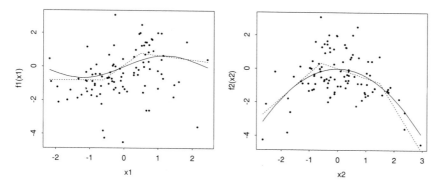

FIGURE 9.14. A simulated example of an additive model. The observed data, the underlying curve components, and the fits are displayed by dots, solid curves, and dotted curves, respectively.

To examine the performance of model (9.38), we rewrite it as two additive components as follows:

$$f_1(x_1) = -0.8 - 1.73(x_1 - 0.48)^+ + 1.48(x_1 + 0.61)^+,$$
$$f_2(x_2) = 1.25 + 1.5x_2 - 2.06(x_2 + 0.6)^+ - 2.21(x_2 - 1.49)^+,$$

where the intercepts were roughly guessed by splitting 0.45. Figure 9.14 plots the observed data points, and the underlying and the fitted components of the model. Although not always, in the present case, the structures of the underlying components are well preserved in the MARS fit.

Example 9.4 *An Interactive Model.*

In the previous examples, we did not consider interaction terms in the underlying functions, nor did we consider nuisance predictors that play no role in the model. To challenge the MARS algorithm, let us allow a second-order interaction term and two nuisance predictors in a hypothetical model.

We took the underlying function to be

$$\frac{1}{20}\exp(4x_1) - x_2\exp(2x_2 - x_3)$$

and drew the additive noise from the standard normal distribution. The predictors x_1 to x_5 were generated independently from the uniform distribution on [0,1]. The sample size was chosen to be 150.

When the MARS model is restricted to be additive, we obtained

$$-0.58 - 2.07x_2 - 8.61(x_2 - 0.716)^+ + 5.71(x_1 - 0.547)^+ + 1.13x_3 \quad (9.39)$$

as the final choice with a GCV value of 1.44. In contrast, if the model is allowed to include the second-order interaction terms, we selected

$$-0.0025 - 3.22x_2 - 8.67(x_2 - 0.716)^+ + 5.50(x_1 - 0.547)^+ + 2.37x_2x_3 \tag{9.40}$$

with a GCV value of 1.38. Models (9.39) and (9.40) are similar, but they differ in the critical interaction term. The latter is slightly favorable in terms of the GCV value. Also, it is noteworthy to mention that model (9.40) was selected again when the third-order interaction terms were permitted in the candidate models.

So far, MARS models appear to be capable of capturing the underlying function structure. We should be aware of the fact that the algorithm can be fooled easily. Note that the five predictors, x_1 to x_5, were generated independently. What happens if we observe $z = x_2 + x_3$, not x_3? Theoretically, this does not affect the information in the data. If we took the difference $z - x_2$ as a new predictor prior to the use of the MARS algorithm, we would arrive at the same model. If we use z directly along with the other predictors, the new underlying model becomes

$$\frac{1}{20}\exp(4x_1) - x_2\exp(3x_2 - z).$$

The fitted model is

$$0.11 - 2.70x_2 - 9.89(x_2 - 0.716)^+ + 5.50(x_1 - 0.547)^+ + +2.57(z - 1.145)^+.$$

Although $(z - 1.145)^+$ can be viewed as some sort of interaction between x_2 and x_3, we do not see an interaction between x_2 and z as being interpretable as the underlying model. This is due partially to the high correlation between x_2 and z (the empirical value is 0.73). Perhaps it is too much to ask; nevertheless, it is prudent to scrutinize the predictors first before getting into the MARS algorithm. For example, simple principal component analyses among the predictors is helpful, especially in the presence of collinearity.

Example 9.5 *MARS Model for Birth Weight*

Now we revisit the analysis of birth weight for the data from the Yale Pregnancy Outcome Study, as was reported in Section 9.1. We use the same variable names as previously defined in Table 2.1 and Section 3.2. When the model is restricted to be additive, we cumulate 29 terms in the forward step in the order z_5, x_9, $(x_9 - 9.2)^+$, x_{15}, $(x_{15} - 1.14)^+$, x_{11}, $(x_{11} - 4.93)^+$, z_{10}, x_{14}, $(x_{14} - 77.1)^+$, x_6, $(x_6 - 14.67)^+$, z_6, z_{11}, x_1, $(x_1, -34.11)^+$, $(x_6 - 25)^+$, $(x_6 - 26)^+$, $(x_6 - 20.74)^+$, $(x_{14} - 160.5)^+$, $(x_1, -42)^+$, $(x_{11} - 8)^+$, $(x_6 - 24)^+$, $(x_{15} - 6)^+$, $(x_{15} - 5)^+$, $(x_{15} - 2)^+$, $(x_1, -38.28)^+$, $(x_1, -36.53)^+$, and $(x_{11} - 5.45)^+$. From these basis functions, the backward step selects 9 terms: z_5,

x_9, $(x_9 - 9.2)^+$, x_{15}, $(x_{15} - 1.14)^+$, $(x_{11} - 4.93)^+$, z_{10}, $(x_6 - 25)^+$, and $(x_6 - 26)^+$. It does not appear particularly meaningful to keep the last two terms in our final model, because they are hardly different from a practical point of view. Thus, the last one is removed. To make the interpretation more straightforward, we change the cutoff values for x_9, x_{11}, and x_{15}, from 9.2, 4.93, and 1.14 to 9, 5, and 1, respectively. After these steps of computer selection and manual adjustment, we arrive at the following model:

$$3141 + 296.4z_5 - 21.7x_9 + 21.7(x_9 - 9)^+ + 111x_{15}$$
$$-88.6(x_{15} - 1)^+ - 102.9(x_{11} - 5)^+ - 276.3z_{10} - 414.1(x_6 - 25)^+, \quad (9.41)$$

which is the mathematical expression of Figure 9.2.

10
Analysis of Longitudinal Data

In health-related studies, researchers often collect data from the same unit (or subject) repeatedly over time. Measurements may be taken at different times for different subjects. These are called longitudinal studies. Diggle, Liang, and Zeger (1994) offer an excellent exposition of the issues related to the design of such studies and the analysis of longitudinal data. They also provide many interesting examples of data. We refer to their book for a thorough treatment of the topic. The purpose of this chapter is to introduce the methods based on recursive partitioning and to compare the analyses of longitudinal data using different approaches.

10.1 Infant Growth Curves

The data for this example were collected from a retrospective study by Dr. John Leventhal and his colleagues at Yale University School of Medicine, New Haven, Connecticut. Their primary aim was to study the risk factors during pregnancy that may lead to the maltreatment of infants after birth such as physical and sexual abuse. The investigators recruited 298 children born at Yale–New Haven Hospital after reviewing the medical records for all women who had deliveries from September 1, 1989, through September 30, 1990. Detailed eligibility criteria have been reported previously elsewhere such as Wasserman and Leventhal (1993) and Stier et al. (1993). The major concern underlying the sample selection was the ascertainment of cocaine exposure. Two groups of infants were included: those whose

138   10. Analysis of Longitudinal Data

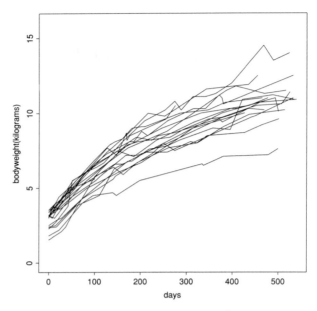

FIGURE 10.1. Growth curves of body weights for 20 representative infants

mothers were regular cocaine users and those whose mothers were clearly not cocaine users. The group membership was classified from the infants' log of toxicology screens and their mothers' obstetric records. In addition, efforts have been made to match the unexposed newborns with the exposed ones for date of birth, medical insurance, mother's parity, age, and timing of the first prenatal visit. The question of our concern is whether a mother's cocaine use has a significant effect on the growth of her infant.

After birth, the infants were brought back to see their pediatricians. At each visit, body weight, height, and head circumference were recorded. Figure 10.1 shows the growth curves of body weights for twenty randomly chosen children.

Figure 10.1 suggests that the variability of weight increases as children grow. Thus, we need to deal with this accelerating variability while modeling the growth curves. In Section 10.5.5 we will explain the actual process of fitting these data. At the moment, we go directly to the result of analysis reported in Zhang (1999) and put on the table what the adaptive spline model can offer in analyzing longitudinal data.

Using mother's cocaine use, infant's gender, gestational age, and race (White or Black) as covariates, Zhang (1999) identified the following model,

$$\hat{f}(\mathbf{x}) = 0.744 + 0.029d - 0.0092(d-120)^+ - 0.0059(d-200)^+ \\ + (g_a - 28)^+ \{0.2 + 0.0005d - 0.0007(d-60)^+ - 0.0009(d-490)^+\} \\ + s\{-0.0026d + 0.0022(d-120)^+\}, \qquad (10.1)$$

where d stands for infant's age in days and g_a for gestational age in weeks. The variable s is the indicator for gender: 1 for girls and 0 for boys. The absence of mother's cocaine use in model (10.1) is a sign against its prominence. Nonetheless, we will reexamine this factor later.

According to model (10.1), the velocity of growth lessens as a child matures. Beyond this common-sense knowledge, model (10.1) defines several interesting phases among which the velocity varies. Note that the knots for age are 60, 120, 200, and 490 days, which are about 2, 4, 8, and 16 months. In other words, as the velocity decreases, its duration doubles. This insight cannot be readily revealed by traditional methods. Furthermore, girls grow slower soon after birth, but start to catch up after four months. Gestational age affects birth weight, as immense evidence has shown. It also influences the growth dynamics. In particular, a more mature newborn tends to grow faster at first, but later experiences a slower growth as opposed to a less mature newborn. Finally, it is appealing that model (10.1) mathematically characterizes the infant growth pattern even without imposing any prior knowledge. This characterization can provide an empirical basis for further refinement of the growth pattern with expert knowledge as well as assessment of other factors of interest.

10.2 The Notation and a General Model

To analyze longitudinal data, first we need to formulate them into a general statistical framework. To this end, some notation is inevitable. Suppose that we have recruited n subjects into a longitudinal study. Measurements are repeatedly taken for every subject over a number of occasions (sometimes referred to as visits or examinations).

Table 10.1 provides an abstract representation of the data such as those plotted in Figure 10.1. To simplify the presentation, we restrict all subjects to have the same number of occasions q in the table. For subject i at occasion j, $x_{k,ij}$ and Y_{ij} are respectively the measurement of the kth covariate

TABLE 10.1. Longitudinal Data Configuration

Subject	Occasion (visit or examination)		
	1	$\cdots$	q
1	$t_{11}, x_{1,11}, \cdots, x_{p,11}, Y_{11}$	$\cdots$	$t_{1q}, x_{1,1q}, \cdots, x_{p,1q}, Y_{1q}$
$\vdots$	$\vdots$		$\vdots$
i	$t_{i1}, x_{1,i1}, \cdots, x_{p,i1}, Y_{i1}$	$\cdots$	$t_{iq}, x_{1,iq}, \cdots, x_{p,iq}, Y_{iq}$
$\vdots$	$\vdots$		$\vdots$
n	$t_{n1}, x_{1,n1}, \cdots, x_{p,n1}, Y_{n1}$	$\cdots$	$t_{nq}, x_{1,nq}, \cdots, x_{p,nq}, Y_{nq}$

Reproduced from Table 1 of Zhang (1997)

x_k ($k = 1, \ldots, p$) and the observed value of the response Y at measurement time t_{ij} ($j = 1, \ldots, q, i = 1, \ldots, n$). In the growth curve data, we have four ($p = 4$) covariates in addition to age (measurement time t) of visits. Birth weight is the outcome variable Y.

The problem of interest is to model the relationship of Y to the measurement time, t, and the p covariates, x_1 to x_p, namely, to establish the relationship

$$Y_{ij} = f(t_{ij}, x_{1,ij}, \ldots, x_{p,ij}) + e_{ij}, \quad (10.2)$$

where f is an unknown function, e_{ij} is the error term, $j = 1, \ldots, q$, and $i = 1, \ldots, n$. Estimating model (10.2) such as the derivation of model (10.1) is imperative for addressing scientific questions for which the data are collected.

Model (10.2) differs from a usual multivariate regression model, e.g., (9.1), in that e_{ij} ($j = 1, \ldots, q$) has an autocorrelation structure Σ_i within the same subject i. As will be defined below, the specification of Σ_i varies from a parametric approach to a nonparametric one.

10.3 Mixed-Effects Models

Mixed-effects models are commonly used to analyze longitudinal data; see, e.g., Crowder and Hand (1990, Ch. 6) and Laird and Ware (1982). They assume that

$$Y_{ij} = \sum_{k=0}^{p} \beta_k x_{k,ij} + \sum_{k=0}^{r} \nu_{ki} z_{k,ij} + \epsilon_{ij}, \quad (10.3)$$

where the β's are unknown parameters, $\boldsymbol{\nu}_i = (\nu_{1i}, \ldots, \nu_{pi})'$ is a p-dimensional random vector, $\boldsymbol{\epsilon}_i = (\epsilon_{i1}, \ldots, \epsilon_{ip})'$ is a p-dimensional vector of measurement errors, and for convenience, t_{ij} is replaced with $x_{0,ij}$. The vector $\boldsymbol{\nu}_i$ reflects the random fluctuation of subject i toward the population, and it is referred to as random coefficients, coupled with random effects z_1 to z_r. The specification of random effect factors has to be decided on a case-by-case basis.

Model (10.3) is called a mixed-effects model or simply a mixed model in light of the fact that the model facilitates both fixed-effect parameters β and random-effect parameters $\boldsymbol{\nu}_i$. Sometimes, model (10.3) is also referred to as two-stage linear model because of the hierarchal assumptions as delineated below.

The first stage describes the distribution for $\boldsymbol{\epsilon}_i$ within the same individual, and the second stage takes into account the across-individual variations expressed through $\boldsymbol{\nu}_i$. Specifically, we assume, in the first stage, that

$$\boldsymbol{\epsilon}_i \sim N(\mathbf{0}, R_i), \ i = 1, \ldots, n, \quad (10.4)$$

10.3 Mixed-Effects Models

and in the second stage that

$$\boldsymbol{\nu}_i \sim N(\mathbf{0}, G), \quad i = 1, \ldots, n, \tag{10.5}$$

and $\boldsymbol{\nu}_i$ and $\boldsymbol{\epsilon}_i$ are independent, $i = 1, \ldots, n$. Moreover, we assume that anything between two individuals is independent of each other.

We can regard model (10.3) as a specific case of model (10.2) in the sense that

$$f(t_{ij}, x_{1,ij}, \ldots, x_{p,ij}) = \sum_{k=0}^{p} \beta_k x_{k,ij}$$

and

$$e_{ij} = \sum_{k=0}^{p} \nu_{ki} x_{k,ij} + \epsilon_{ij},$$

$j = 1, \ldots, q$, $i = 1, \ldots, n$. Let $\mathbf{y}_i = (Y_{i1}, \ldots, Y_{iq})'$. Then assumptions (10.4) and (10.5) imply that

$$\mathbb{E}\{\mathbf{y}_i\} = X_i \boldsymbol{\beta}, \quad \Sigma_i = \text{Cov}\{\mathbf{y}_i\} = X_i G X_i' + R_i,$$

where X_i is the design matrix for individual i, i.e.,

$$X_i = \begin{pmatrix} x_{0,i1} & \cdots & x_{p,i1} \\ \vdots & \vdots & \vdots \\ x_{0,ij} & \cdots & x_{p,ij} \\ \vdots & \vdots & \vdots \\ x_{0,iq} & \cdots & x_{p,iq} \end{pmatrix}, \quad i = 1, \ldots, n.$$

What are the essential steps in applying model (10.3) for the analysis of longitudinal data? A convenient approach to carry out the computation is the use of PROC MIXED in the SAS package. One tricky step is the specification of random effects. It requires knowledge of the particular study design and objective. See Kleinbaum et al. (1988, Ch. 17) for general guidelines. Following this step, it remains for us to specify the classes of covariance structures R_i in (10.4) and G in (10.5).

In practice, R_i is commonly chosen as a diagonal matrix; for example, $R_i = \sigma_1^2 I$; here I is an identity matrix. The resulting model is referred to as a conditional independence model. In other words, the measurements within the same individuals are independent after removing the random-effect components. In applications, a usual choice for G is $\sigma_2^2 I$. The dimension of this identity matrix is omitted, and obviously it should conform with G. The subscripts of σ remind us of the stage in which these covariance matrices take part.

There are many other choices for covariance matrices. A thorough list of options is available from SAS Online Help. Diggle, Liang, and Zeger (1994) devote an excellent chapter on the understanding of covariance structure

10. Analysis of Longitudinal Data

TABLE 10.2. A Sample SAS Program for Analyzing Longitudinal Data
```
data   one;
infile 'infant.dat';
input  infantID race npp mage gender coc ga age wtkg;
eage = exp(age/100.);
run;
proc mixed;
    model wtkg = coc gender|age gender|eage ga|age ga|eage;
    repeated /type=ar(1) subject=person;
run;
```

for longitudinal data. Ironically, the simplest choice is still taken for granted in most of the applications. We will offer a general and brief guideline for estimating the covariance structure and also illustrate use of some graphical approaches in real applications.

For comparison, let us analyze the infant growth data with **PROC MIXED** in SAS. The initial model includes eight main-effect terms [race, the number of previous pregnancies (coded as **npp**), mother's age at delivery (**mage**), mother's cocaine use (**coc**), gestational age (**gage**), child's gender, child's age at a visit, and an exponential transformation of the child's age] and four interaction terms (gender and gestational age by age and the transformation of age). These variables are specified in the **model** statement in Table 10.2 as fixed effects. Subject number is the only random effect. In addition, the covariance is set to have an AR(1) structure (see, e.g., Box et al., 1994, p. 58) in the **repeated** statement.

Using the backward stepwise deletion, we conclude with the following model:

$$-4.0 + 0.18c + 0.194g_a - 0.115s + 0.02d - 0.0008sd$$
$$+0.006 \exp(d/100) - 0.0005 g_a \exp(d/100), \qquad (10.6)$$

where c denotes mother's cocaine use and the other variables are the same as those in model (10.1). Most of the p-values are below the 0.05 level except for s (child's gender) and $\exp(d/100)$, which are at the 0.2 level and are kept to accompany the second-order interaction terms. From this model, mother's cocaine use manifests itself with a marginal significance of 0.03.

Broadly, model (10.6) gives rise to similar conclusions to what the spline model (10.1) does. However, model (10.1) fits the data better than model (10.6). An important point to remember is that considering the transformations and interactions for the predictors in a mixed model is usually tedious and time-consuming. The spline model may offer a much quicker and sometimes more realistic look into the data structure. We recommend using spline models first and refining them based on expert knowledge.

10.4 Semiparametric Models

As in multiple linear regression, the linear assumption in mixed-effects models makes it inconvenient to explore nonlinear time trends. To accommodate general time trends for longitudinal data, Diggle, Liang, and Zeger (1994, p. 111) and Zeger and Diggle (1994) presented the following semiparametric model:

$$Y_{ij} = \beta_0 + \sum_{k=1}^{p} \beta_k x_{k,ij} + \mu(t_{ij}) + e_i(t_{ij}), \qquad (10.7)$$

where μ is an unspecified smooth function. Unlike mixed-effects models, the semiparametric model (10.7) includes a practically arbitrary time trend. Note also that the error term in model (10.7) is explicitly expressed as a function of time, and it corresponds to the sum of two parts in model (10.3): individual random effects and measurement errors. Precisely, Diggle et al. assume that $\{Y_{ij}(t), t \in R\}$ for $i = 1, \ldots, n$ are independent copies of a stationary Gaussian process, $\{Y(t)\}$, with variance σ^2 and correlation function $\rho(\Delta)$. This means that for any time points $t_1, \ldots, t_k$ and an increment Δ,

$$(Y(t_1), \ldots, Y(t_k)) \text{ and } (Y(t_1 + \Delta), \ldots, w(Y_k + \Delta))$$

have the same multivariate normal distribution, and the correlation between $Y(t)$ and $Y(t + \Delta)$ is $\rho(\Delta)$. Examples of $\rho(\Delta)$ are

$$\exp(-\alpha \Delta) \text{ and } \exp(-\alpha \Delta^2), \qquad (10.8)$$

where α needs to be estimated from the data.

As an example of the back-fitting algorithm of Hastie and Tibshirani (1990), Diggle, Liang, and Zeger (1994) proposed to fit model (10.7) in three steps: (a) Find a kernel estimate of μ for a given estimate $\hat{\boldsymbol{\beta}}$ using the residuals model

$$Y_{ij} - \hat{\beta}_0 - \sum_{k=1}^{p} \hat{\beta}_k x_{k,ij} = \mu(t_{ij}) + e_i(t_{ij}). \qquad (10.9)$$

(b) Update the estimate $\hat{\boldsymbol{\beta}}$ from the residuals $r_{ij} = Y_{ij} - \hat{\mu}(t_{ij})$ using generalized least squares,

$$\hat{\boldsymbol{\beta}} = (X'\Psi^{-1}X)^{-1}X'\Psi^{-1}\mathbf{r}, \qquad (10.10)$$

where $X = (X_1', \ldots, X_n')'$, $\mathbf{r}$ is the concatenate vector of r_{ij} for $i = 1, \ldots, n$ and $j = 1, \ldots, q$, and Ψ is a block diagonal covariance matrix with the ith block being the covariance matrix Σ_i. (c) Repeat steps (a) and (b) for convergence, which typically takes a few iterations.

We will not discuss how to obtain a kernel estimate of μ required in step (a) and refer to Hart and Wehrly (1986), Rice and Silverman (1991), Truong (1991), and Altman (1992). It is important to point out, though, that $\hat{\mu}$ must be computed numerically and cannot be expressed in a closed form unless adaptive splines are adopted.

Step (b) involves a covariance matrix that by itself is unknown. With a simple choice of $\rho(\Delta)$ it is usually not difficult to estimate Ψ and β simultaneously.

Further details in the implementation and theoretical properties of this method are available in Zeger and Diggle (1994) and Moyeed and Diggle (1994).

10.5 Adaptive Spline Models

The mixed-effects model (10.3) and the semiparametric model (10.7) provide very useful means to model building of longitudinal data. It is also important for us to realize some limitations of these models and seek an alternative.

Both the mixed-effects models and the semiparametric models are parametric with respect to the covariates. Hence, they have limited flexibilities for including transformations of, and interactions among, covariates.

Semiparametric models allow for a general time trend, but they can be handicapped in the presence of interactive effects between time and some of the covariates. If the covariates are categorical, it is possible to fit different trends at different levels of the variables. Obviously, the success of this attempt depends severely on the sample size available. When a covariate is of continuous scale, the solution is not apparent.

To overcome the limitations of the mixed-effects models and the semiparametric models posed above, Zhang (1997) considered a functionally nonparametric model

$$Y_{ij} = f(t_{ij}, x_{1,ij}, \ldots, x_{p,ij}) + e_i(\mathbf{x}_{*,ij}, t_{ij}), \qquad (10.11)$$

where f is an unknown smooth function and the $\mathbf{x}_*$ indicates some dependency of the error term on the explanatory variables. This dependency will be clarified in Section 10.5.2. To avoid technicality, we assume again that $e_i(\mathbf{x}_{*,ij}, t)$ is a high-dimensional stationary Gaussian process. Model (10.11) can be regarded as a generalization of the semiparametric model (10.7). It distinguishes itself from the general model (10.2) by explicitly expressing the error term as a function of time.

The discussion below is mostly adopted from Zhang (1997), where he proposed multivariate adaptive splines for the analysis of longitudinal data (MASAL).

The goal of MASAL is to fit model (10.11). It requires three broad steps: (a) Given a covariance structure for $e_i(\mathbf{x}_{*,ij}, t_{ij})$, find an adaptive spline estimate of f using the ideas introduced in Chapter 9. (b) Update the estimate of the covariance structure from the residuals, $r_{ij} = Y_{ij} - \hat{f}_{ij}$, $i = 1, \ldots, n$ and $j = 1, \ldots, q$. (c) Repeat steps (a) and (b) until convergence.

These three steps are similar to those stated in the previous section. Crowder and Hand (1990, p. 73) vividly described it as a see-saw algorithm. As a matter of fact, if every step of the estimation is based on maximizing a certain likelihood function, this three-step algorithm is a "generalized" version of the method called restricted maximum likelihood estimation (REML), which was introduced by Patterson and Thompson (1971) to estimate variance components in a general linear model and has recently been applied in the longitudinal data setting (e.g., McGilchrist and Cullis, 1991). The merits of the REML estimators in the context of mixed models have been explored by many authors (e.g., Cressie and Lahiri, 1993, and Richardson and Welsh, 1994). It is reasonable to hope that some of the important properties of REML estimators also hold for the MASAL estimators.

Section 10.5.1 describes the implementation of step (a), and Section 10.5.2 addresses that of step (b).

10.5.1 Known Covariance Structure

When Σ_i's (or equivalently the block diagonal matrix Ψ) are given, we employ the weighted sum of squares (WSS) as the measure of goodness-of-fit for model (10.11). That is,

$$WSS(f) = (\mathbf{y} - \mathbf{f})'\Psi^{-1}(\mathbf{y} - \mathbf{f}), \quad (10.12)$$

where

$$\mathbf{y} = (\mathbf{y}_1', \ldots, \mathbf{y}_n')' \quad (10.13)$$

and

$$\mathbf{f} = (f(t_{11}, x_{1,11}, \ldots, x_{p,11}), \ldots, f(t_{ij}, x_{1,ij}, \ldots, x_{p,ij}),$$
$$\ldots, f(t_{nq}, x_{1,nq}, \ldots, x_{p,nq}))'.$$

From a structural point of view, the forward algorithm in Section 9.4 and the backward algorithm in Section 9.5 still apply to the present case. The difference resides in the realization of every step. Here, we emphasize the differences and difficulties and refer to Zhang (1997) for the details.

Obviously, the source of differences is the autocorrelation of the residual term in model (10.11). When the covariance matrix Ψ is assumed to be known, we can transform $\mathbf{y}$ so that the transformed observations are independent. In other words, we work on

$$\mathbf{z} = \Psi^{-\frac{1}{2}}\mathbf{y}, \quad (10.14)$$

where $\Psi^{-\frac{1}{2}}\Psi^{-\frac{1}{2}} = \Psi^{-1}$.

If model (10.11) were a linear model, the transformed data would lead to a weighted least squares estimate of f similar to (10.10). Unfortunately, model (10.11) is not linear, and we will see why the nonlinearity deserves special attention.

Recall the construction of an initial MARS model (9.10). The first and also critical step in the forward algorithm is to find the best knot $\hat{\tau}$ associated with a covariate x_k such that the WSS in (10.12) is minimized when $\mathbf{f}$ is chosen to be of the form

$$\mathbf{f} = \beta_0 \mathbf{1} + \beta_1 \mathbf{x}_{k\cdot\cdot} + \beta_2 (\mathbf{x}_{k\cdot\cdot} - \tau \mathbf{1})^+, \tag{10.15}$$

where

$$\mathbf{x}_{k\cdot\cdot} = (x_{k,11}, \ldots, x_{k,1q}, \ldots, x_{k,i1}, \ldots, x_{k,iq}, \ldots, x_{k,n1}, \ldots, x_{k,nq})'.$$

This is the concatenate vector for all values of predictor x_k.

With the specification in (10.15) and the transformation in (10.14), model (10.11) becomes the following regression model:

$$\mathbf{z} = \beta_0 \Psi^{-\frac{1}{2}}\mathbf{1} + \beta_1 \Psi^{-\frac{1}{2}}\mathbf{x}_{k\cdot\cdot} + \beta_2 \Psi^{-\frac{1}{2}}\mathbf{b}(\tau) + \Psi^{-\frac{1}{2}}\mathbf{e}, \tag{10.16}$$

where $\mathbf{b}(\tau) = (\mathbf{x}_{k\cdot\cdot} - \tau\mathbf{1})^+$. Finding $\hat{\tau}$ is not difficult, but it is challenging to find the solution in the least possible time. Speed is a concern because the same algorithm is used many times.

What are potential impediments of designing such a desirable algorithm? First, the WSS in (10.12) needs to be expressed as a simple function of τ. Second, we ought to be able to calculate the WSS efficiently as we search $\hat{\tau}$ through the observed range of x_k. We have demonstrated that these are possible in Chapter 9, where Ψ is essentially an identity matrix. The problem in model (10.16) is that

$$\Psi^{-\frac{1}{2}}\mathbf{b}(\tau) \neq (\Psi^{-\frac{1}{2}}\mathbf{x}_{k\cdot\cdot} - \Psi^{-\frac{1}{2}}\mathbf{1})^+,$$

due to the nonlinearity. We refer to Zhang (1997) for the derivation of an explicit and efficient algorithm for finding $\hat{\tau}$.

10.5.2 Unknown Covariance Structure

In practical problems, it is virtually always the case that the covariance structure is unknown. We need to estimate both the covariance structure Ψ and fixed-effect function f, alternately. In the preceding section, we explained how to estimate the fixed-effect function using adaptive splines for any given covariance structure. The question now is how to update the covariance structure when the function is estimated.

For any estimate $\hat{f}$ of function f we can calculate the residuals $r_{ij} = Y_{ij} - \hat{f}_{ij}$, where $\hat{f}_{ij}$ is the estimated function value for the ith subject at occasion j, $j = 1, \ldots, q$, $i = 1, \ldots, n$. Note that one of the assumptions in model (10.11) is the normality of the residuals. Thus, the question is really, How do we estimate the covariance matrix of a q-variate normal distribution based on the observed data?

The answer is relatively easy if q is much smaller than n, because the sample covariance matrix would serve as an estimate of the covariance matrix. This results in the so-called unstructured estimate of the covariance matrix. In many applications, however, q is not small relative to n, and hence it is often desirable to impose certain restrictions on the underlying covariance structure, e.g., the compound symmetry structure:

$$\Sigma_i = \sigma^2 \begin{pmatrix} 1 & \rho & \cdots & \rho \\ \rho & 1 & \cdots & \rho \\ \vdots & \vdots & \vdots & \vdots \\ \rho & \rho & \cdots & \rho \end{pmatrix}. \tag{10.17}$$

This covariance matrix is sometimes referred to as uniform correlation (Diggle, Liang, and Zeger, 1994, p. 56).

When the times are equally spaced, the following stationary form is also a reasonable choice for Σ_i

$$\begin{pmatrix} \sigma^2 & \sigma_1 & \cdots & \sigma_{q-2} & \sigma_{q-1} \\ \sigma_1 & \sigma^2 & \cdots & \sigma_{q-3} & \sigma_{q-2} \\ \vdots & \vdots & \vdots & \vdots & \vdots \\ \sigma_{q-2} & \sigma_{q-3} & \cdots & \sigma^2 & \sigma_1 \\ \sigma_{q-1} & \sigma_{q-2} & \cdots & \sigma_1 & \sigma^2 \end{pmatrix}. \tag{10.18}$$

In general, the Σ_i's are assumed to depend on a common parameter vector $\boldsymbol{\theta}$ (Laird and Ware, 1982). In the case of compound symmetry, $\boldsymbol{\theta} = (\sigma^2, \rho)$. For the stationary form, $\boldsymbol{\theta} = (\sigma^2, \sigma_1, \ldots, \sigma_{q-1})$.

It is natural to wonder whether these ad hoc structures are appropriate and whether there are general guidelines in making such a decision. These issues are always puzzling in the analysis of longitudinal data regardless of the analytic methods. To get some insights into these issues, let us follow the discussion in Diggle, Liang, and Zeger (1994, Chapter 5).

To select a reasonable covariance structure, we must first understand the attributes of the covariance structure. Although not necessarily exclusive, three major underlying stochastic processes usually underlie the covariance structure, and they are random effects, serial correlation, and measurement error. In general, we assume that these three potential sources of uncertainty function in an additive manner:

$$e_{ij} = \mathbf{x}'_{*,ij}\mathbf{u} + w(t_{ij}) + \epsilon_{ij}, \tag{10.19}$$

where the three terms represent, respectively, random effects, serial correlation, and measurement error.

In (10.19), **u** is a vector of Gaussian variables with mean zero and covariance matrix G, corresponding to the random effects $\mathbf{x}_{*,ij}$. In some studies, for example, the response profile of one subject may have a greater uncertainty than those of others. Hopefully, this difference in the variability can be characterized through a subset, or transformations, of the original p covariates.

Although the extent may vary, it is conceivable that some lasting variabilities within the same subject may manifest themselves through time as we repeatedly collect measurements. In other words, the response profile of one subject is likely to be an autocorrelated time series. This autocorrelation is reflected by $w(t)$. We assume that $w(t)$ is a stationary Gaussian process with mean zero, covariance σ_2^2, and correlation function $\rho(\Delta)$.

Finally, measurement errors arise in virtually any study. Their magnitude may depend on the quality of equipment, the experience of the investigators, etc. In (10.19), ϵ_{ij} denotes these "isolated" measurement errors. It is common to assume that the ϵ_{ij}'s are independently identically distributed as $N(0, \sigma_1^2)$.

The synthesis of (10.19) with the associated assumptions implies that

$$\Sigma_i = \text{Cov}(\mathbf{e}_i) = X'_{*,i} G X_{*,i} + \sigma_2^2 H + \sigma_1^2 I_q, \qquad (10.20)$$

where $X_{*,i}$ is the design matrix from the ith subject restricted to the random effects only, and H is the autocorrelation matrix

$$\begin{pmatrix} 1 & \rho(t_2 - t_1) & \cdots & \rho(t_q - t_1) \\ \vdots & \vdots & \vdots & \vdots \\ \rho(t_q - t_1) & \rho(t_q - t_2) & \cdots & 1 \end{pmatrix}. \qquad (10.21)$$

Here, we assume that $t_{ij} = t_j$ for $j = 1, \ldots, q$ and $i = 1, \ldots, n$. Two popular choices of ρ are given in (10.8). To avoid being overly complex, we may restrict G in (10.20) to have compound symmetry. In this regard, it is important to note that a covariance structure with compound symmetry may not necessarily be apparent from the observed data. To demonstrate this point, we simulated 100 vectors of 5-dimensional normal random variables with variance 4 and uniform correlation 0.2. The sample covariance matrices from two experiments are

$$\begin{pmatrix} 4.35 & 1.00 & 1.08 & 0.95 & 1.05 \\ 1.00 & 4.28 & 1.20 & 1.15 & 1.55 \\ 1.08 & 1.20 & 3.44 & 0.44 & 1.53 \\ 0.95 & 1.15 & 0.44 & 4.19 & 0.87 \\ 1.05 & 1.55 & 1.53 & 0.87 & 3.90 \end{pmatrix}, \begin{pmatrix} 3.96 & 0.60 & 1.16 & 0.81 & 0.54 \\ 0.60 & 4.39 & 0.82 & 0.32 & 0.88 \\ 1.16 & 0.82 & 4.06 & 0.25 & 0.19 \\ 0.81 & 0.32 & 0.25 & 3.59 & 0.58 \\ 0.54 & 0.88 & 0.19 & 0.58 & 3.31 \end{pmatrix}.$$

Visually, they do not seem to possess compound symmetry even though the data that were generated follow it. Therefore, in practice, it may not be wise to abandon the use of compound symmetry unless there is a clear trend in the covariance structure that contradicts it.

10.5 Adaptive Spline Models

TABLE 10.3. Variables in the Simulation

Variable	Characteristics	Specification
t	Time	1 to q
x_1	Baseline Covariate	Uniform [0,1]
x_2	Baseline Covariate	Uniform [0,1]
x_3	Baseline Covariate	Uniform [0,1]
x_4	Time-Dependent Covariate	Uniform [0,1]
x_5	Time-Dependent Covariate	Uniform [0,1]
x_6	Time-Dependent Covariate	Uniform [0,1]
Y	Response Variable	The model (10.11)

Reproduced from Table 2 of Zhang (1997).

After we set up the basic structure for Σ_i, we can estimate its parameters by maximizing the reduced log-likelihood function for Ψ,

$$l_r(\Psi) = -\log(|\Psi|) - (\mathbf{y} - \hat{\mathbf{f}})'\Psi^{-1}(\mathbf{y} - \hat{\mathbf{f}}), \qquad (10.22)$$

where Ψ is the block diagonal matrix with Σ_i's along the diagonal.

10.5.3 A Simulated Example

In this section we demonstrate the use of MASAL with a simulated data set. Table 10.3 lists the variables involved in the simulation, including time t, response Y, three baseline covariates x_1 to x_3, and three time-dependent covariates x_4 to x_6.

Example 10.1 Consider a 5-dimensional function

$$f(t, \mathbf{x}) = 10t + 10\sin(x_1 x_4 \pi) + 20(x_2 - \frac{1}{2})^2 + 5x_5. \qquad (10.23)$$

This is one of the functional structures studied by Zhang (1997). A few points are worth mentioning. First, x_3 and x_6 are not in f, and hence they are noise (or nuisance) predictors. Second, the function includes both linear and nonlinear terms. Lastly, it also has additive and multiplicative terms.

The data simulation process is as follows. We choose $n = 100$ and $q = 5$. The observations for Y are obtained from model (10.11). The measurement error is generated from a 5-dimensional normal distribution with a covariance matrix whose diagonal elements equal 4 and off-diagonal elements 0.8. The sample covariance matrices from the signal (or the true function) and the noise are respectively

$$\begin{pmatrix} 4.97 & 0.42 & 0.29 & 1.08 & 1.12 \\ 0.42 & 4.20 & 1.15 & 0.59 & 1.21 \\ 0.29 & 1.15 & 3.83 & 0.75 & 1.16 \\ 1.08 & 0.59 & 0.75 & 3.89 & 1.29 \\ 1.12 & 1.21 & 1.16 & 1.29 & 4.33 \end{pmatrix}$$

TABLE 10.4. Model Fitting for Example 10.5.3.

Iteration	The Fitted Model	d_c	l_r
1	$3.79 + 9.92t + 27.3x_1x_4 - 21x_1(x_4 - 0.47)^+$ $-61.6(x_1 - 0.53)^+(x_4 - 0.47)^+ - 10.2x_2$ $+12.8(x_2 - 0.43)^+ + 94.7(x_2 - 0.75)^+x_5$ $-107(x_2 - 0.75)^+(x_5 - 0.22)^+ + 5.76x_5$ $+8.13(x_4 - 0.47)^+ - 11.4(x_4 - 0.75)^+x_5$	2091	-1525
2	$3.89 + 9.91t + 28.7x_1x_4 - 14.9(x_1 - 0.6)^+x_4$ $-69.8(x_1 - 0.4)^+(x_4 - 0.53)^+ - 8.55x_2$ $+19.4(x_2 - 0.54)^+ + 5.34x_5$	1	-1190
3	$3.9 + 9.91t + 28.6x_1x_4 - 15(x_1 - 0.6)^+x_4$ $-70(x_1 - 0.4)^+(x_4 - 0.53)^+ - 8.57x_2$ $+19.4(x_2 - 0.54)^+ + 5.37x_5$	0.001	-1189

and

$$\begin{pmatrix} 12.9 & 6.12 & 6.47 & 5.46 & 5.86 \\ 6.12 & 13.7 & 7.50 & 6.42 & 6.90 \\ 6.47 & 7.50 & 16.6 & 5.62 & 5.98 \\ 5.46 & 6.42 & 5.62 & 16.3 & 6.78 \\ 5.86 & 6.90 & 5.98 & 6.78 & 15.3 \end{pmatrix}.$$

These two matrices show that the size of the occasionwise signal-to-noise ratio is in the range of 2.6 to 4.3.

During the fitting, the maximum number of terms is 20, and the highest order of interactions permitted is 2. To examine the change in the iterative model-building process, we report not only the subsequent models in Table 10.4, but also a measure of difference, d_c, between two consecutive covariance matrices and the log-likelihood, l_r, in (10.22).

All information in Table 10.4 (the fitted model, d_c, and l_r) reveals that further continuation of cycling has little effect on the fit. The two nuisance predictors, x_3 and x_6, do not appear in any of the models. The fitted models after the second iteration capture all four terms in the original structure. Let us choose the model in the third iteration as our final model. We see that t and x_5 are included as linear effects with roughly the same coefficients as the true values. The sum $-8.57x_2 + 19.4(x_2 - 0.54)^+$ corresponds to the quadratic term $10(x_2 - \frac{1}{2})^2$ in the true model. The knot 0.54 is close to the underlying center 0.5 of the parabola, and the coefficients match reasonably with the true values. The only multiplicative effects are for x_1 and x_4. The proxy for their sinusoidal function is $28.6x_1x_4 - 15(x_1 - 0.6)^+x_4 - 70(x_1 - 0.4)^+(x_4 - 0.53)$. In Figure 10.2, we compare $10\sin(x_1x_4\pi)$ with

$$28.6x_1x_4 - 15(x_1 - 0.6)^+x_4 - 70(x_1 - 0.4)^+(x_4 - 0.53) \qquad (10.24)$$

along the two diagonal lines $x_1 = x_4$ and $x_1 = 1 - x_4$.

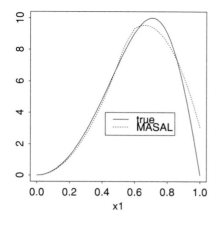
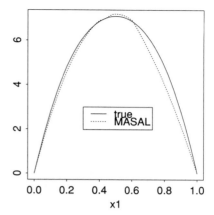

FIGURE 10.2. Comparison of the true $(10\sin(x_1 x_4 \pi))$ and MASAL (10.24) curves along two diagonal lines: $x_1 = x_4$ (left) and $x_1 = 1 - x_4$ (right).

This example demonstrates that the MASAL model is capable of uncovering both the overall and the detailed structure of the underlying model. On the other hand, it is very easy to make the MASAL model fail by increasing the noise level. In that case, we may not have any better alternative.

For comparison, let us see what happens when the mixed-effects model (10.3) is employed. We adopted a backward stepwise procedure by initially including 7 linear terms, t and x_1 to x_6, and their second-order interaction terms. The significance level for including a term in the final model is 0.05. The following model was derived:

$$-0.5 + 10.6t + 9.5x_1 + 4.49x_2 + 13.8x_4 - 1.44tx_4 - 6.4x_1x_4 - 10.2x_2x_4. \tag{10.25}$$

Some aspects of model (10.25) are noteworthy. Firstly, it does not have a quadratic term of x_2 because "we did not know" a priori that we should consider it. Secondly, it excludes the linear term of x_5. Thirdly, it includes two interaction terms tx_4 and x_2x_4 that are not in the true model. Lastly, the interaction term between x_1 and x_4 proves to be significant, but it is difficult from a practical standpoint to consider the nonlinear terms of x_1 and x_4.

In fairness to the mixed-effects model, we fitted the data again by attaching x_2^2 and x_5 to model (10.25). Not surprisingly, they turned out to be significant, but the interaction term x_1x_4 was not. Thus, we lost the true interaction terms while retaining the two false ones. The point is that there is nothing wrong theoretically with the mixed-effects model. We end up with an imprecise model usually because we do not know where we should start from. The present example is a simulation study. The real problems are generally more difficult to deal with. In a word, the importance of the

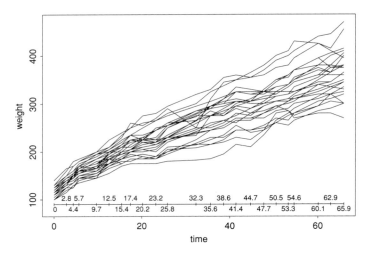

FIGURE 10.3. Body weights of twenty-six cows

mixed-effects model is undeniable, but we also should realistically face its limitations.

10.5.4 Reanalyses of Two Published Data Sets

To explain further the use of MASAL and compare it with that of more standard approaches, we analyze two published data sets.

Example 10.2 *Body Weights of Cows*

The data for this example are taken from Table 5.2 of Diggle, Liang, and Zeger (1994). The outcome measure is the body weights of 26 cows in a 2 by 2 factorial experiment. The body weights of these cows were measured at 23 unequally spaced times over 22 months. Like Diggle et al., we use a rescaled time unit of ten days. Figure 10.3 depicts the growth curves of the cows in the rescaled time as marked under the curves. As in Figure 10.1, the variability of growth curves is greater as the cows gained more weight.

The two factors are presence or absence of iron dosing and of infection with paratuberculosi. The question of clinical interest is the factorial effect on the body weight. These factors determine four factorial groups: control, iron dosing, infection, and iron dosing with infection. We introduce two dummy variables: x_1 as the indicator for iron dosing and x_2 as that for infection. In addition, we use $x_3 = x_1 x_2$ as the interaction between x_1 and x_2.

We will take an analytic strategy different from that of Diggle, Liang, and Zeger (1994, p. 102) in two aspects. First, they took a log-transformation of body weights to stabilize the variance over time. Figure 10.4 displays the sample covariance matrices (the dots) against time for the body weights and their log-transformations. This figure shows that the variance of the transformed weights varies over time with a roughly quadratic trend, as was also noted by Zhang (1997). Therefore, it is not particularly evident that the log-transform indeed stabilized the variance over time. On the other hand, the variance obtained from the original body weights seems to be described well by a Gaussian form in (10.27) below. For these reasons, we will analyze the original body weights, not their log-transformations. As an aside, note that the log-transformation has little effect on the trend of the autocorrelation.

Since the time trend is not their primary interest, Diggle et al. had a clever idea of avoiding fitting the time trend while addressing the major hypothesis. This was made possible by taking a pointwise average of the growth curve for the control group ($x_1 = x_2 = 0$) and then modeling the differences between the weights in other groups and the average of the controls. They assumed quadratic time trends for the differences. Generally speaking, however, it is wise to be aware of the shortcomings of this approach. Twenty-three parameters are needed to derive the average profile for the control group although the actual trend can be fitted well with a fewer number of parameters. As a consequence, the differences may involve a greater variability and eventually could influence the final conclusion. Since MASAL is designed to fit an arbitrary time trend, the differencing is no longer necessary, nor is it desirable. Thus, we will fit directly the body weights based on the two factors and time. This clarifies the second difference between our strategy and that of Diggle et al.

The number of occasions, $q = 23$, is obviously large as opposed to the number of subjects, $n = 26$. It does not make much sense to use an unstructured covariance matrix. Thus, we have to explore the covariance structure before doing any modeling. When we choose a covariance structure, it is clearly important to capture the overall time trend, but it could be counter productive if we devoted too many degrees of freedom in the time trend.

The top two panels in Figure 10.4 display respectively the autocorrelation against the time difference $\Delta_{ij} = t_i - t_j$ (left) and the variance against time (right) on the original weight scale. The time difference Δ will be referred to as lag. The autocorrelation seems to decrease linearly in lag, and the variance behaves as a Gaussian function. Specifically, using the least squares method, we fitted the autocorrelation as a linear function of lag and arrived at

$$\hat{\rho}(\Delta) = 0.94 - 0.0037\Delta. \qquad (10.26)$$

For the variance we have

$$\hat{\sigma}^2(t) = \exp(4.73 + 0.097t - 0.00083t^2). \qquad (10.27)$$

154   10. Analysis of Longitudinal Data

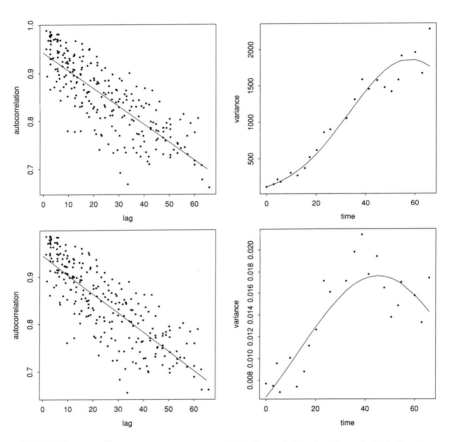

FIGURE 10.4. Covariance structures of body weights (top) and their log transformations (bottom). The dots are the sample estimates, and the solid lines and curves are the least squares fits.

10.5 Adaptive Spline Models

TABLE 10.5. Basis Functions Entered in the Initial Forward Step

Step	Basis function
1	Intercept
2	x_1, x_2, and x_3
3	t and $(t-6)^+$
4	$(t-17.4)^+$
5	$(t-9.7)^+$
6	tx_2 and $(t-23.2)^+ x_2$
7	$(t-17.7)^+ x_2$
8	$(t-4.4)^+ x_2$
9	$(t-25.8)^+$
10	tx_1 and $(t-12.5)^+ x_1$
11	$(t-62.7)^+ x_2$
12	tx_3 and $(t-44.7)^+ x_3$
13	$(t-41.4)^+ x_3$
14	$(t-50.5)^+ x_3$

Following (10.26) and (10.27), we assume that the covariance structure can be characterized by

$$\rho(\Delta) = \phi_1 + \phi_2 \Delta \text{ and } \sigma^2(t) = \exp(\nu_1 + \nu_2 t + \nu_3 t^2). \quad (10.28)$$

Thus, the problem of estimating the covariance structure becomes that of estimating parameters ϕ and ν in (10.28), because the within-subject covariance matrix, Σ_i, is a function of $\rho(\Delta)$ and $\sigma^2(t)$ evaluated at the measurement times.

We first use (10.26) and (10.27) as our initial estimates. In the subsequent iterations, the estimates will be derived from maximizing the log-likelihood (10.22) by holding $\hat{\mathbf{f}}$ fixed. For example, as Table 10.7 shows, the covariance estimates in the second iteration are

$$\hat{\rho}(\Delta) = 0.96 - 0.0078\Delta \text{ and } \hat{\sigma}^2(t) = \exp(5.09 + 0.06t - 0.00045t^2). \quad (10.29)$$

In many applications, data are collected for some specific aims. In this example, for instance, the main interest now is to examine the effect of iron dosing, infection, and their potential interaction on the growth of cows. In such a circumstance, we have nothing to lose by entering the three variables x_1 to x_3 of clinical interest into the MASAL model before the forward step starts to cumulate basis functions. Table 10.5 displays the basis functions in the order they appear during the forward step in the first (initial) iteration.

Holding the 20 terms in Table 10.5 as if they were fixed, we remove one least-significant term at a time. This deletion process gives rise to 19 reduced models, from which we choose the one leading to the smallest

TABLE 10.6. Model Fitting for Body Weights of Cows

Iteration	The Fitted Model	l_r
1	$117 + 9.1t - 6.4(t-6)^+ + 2.5(t-9.7)^+$ $-1.9(t-25.8)^+ - 2.2x_2 t + 2x_2(t-4.4)^+$ $-4.4x_2(t-17.7)^+ + 4.5x_2(t-23.2)^+$	-3197
2	$117 + 9.1t - 6.1(t-5.7)^+ + 2.2(t-9.7)^+$ $-1.9(t-25.8)^+ - 2.3x_2 t + 2.1x_2(t-4.4)^+$ $-4.2x_2(t-17.4)^+ + 4.3x_2(t-23.2)^+$	-3134
3	$117 + 9.1t - 6.1(t-5.7)^+ + 2.2(t-9.7)^+$ $-1.9(t-25.8)^+ - 2.3x_2 t + 2.1x_2(t-4.4)^+$ $-4.2x_2(t-17.4)^+ + 4.3x_2(t-23.2)^+$	-3134

TABLE 10.7. Covariance Estimates

Iteration	Estimated covariance equation
1	$\hat{\rho}(\Delta) = 0.94 - 0.0037\Delta$ $\hat{\sigma}^2(t) = \exp(4.73 + 0.097t - 0.00083t^2)$
2	$\hat{\rho}(\Delta) = 0.96 - 0.0078\Delta$ $\hat{\sigma}^2(t) = \exp(5.09 + 0.06t - 0.00045t^2)$
3	$\hat{\rho}(\Delta) = 0.96 - 0.0079\Delta$ $\hat{\sigma}^2(t) = \exp(5.09 + 0.06t - 0.00045t^2)$

GCV. The selected model in the initial iteration is the first one in Table 10.6. Two subsequently selected models are also given in the same table. Besides, Table 10.7 displays the estimates of the covariance parameters in all iterations. These tables indicate that the fitting process converges at the second iteration. The discrepancy between the second and third iterations is negligible. Thus, we choose the final MASAL as

$$117 + 9.1t - 6.1(t-5.7)^+ + 2.2(t-9.7)^+ - 1.9(t-25.8)^+ \\ -\{2.3t - 2.1(t-4.4)^+ + 4.2(t-17.4)^+ - 4.3(t-23.2)^+\}x_2. \quad (10.30)$$

To evaluate the adequacy of model (10.30), we display the residuals and fitted curves in Figure 10.5. In the left panel, both the residuals and predictions are transformed via the square root of the third-iteration covariance matrix presented in Table 10.7. The separate growth curves on the right-hand side are drawn for infected and uninfected cows. The weights between the two groups were not substantially different for the first half year. However, from the sixth to eighth months, the infected cows had grown much more slowly than had the uninfected ones, causing a difference between the two groups. The magnitude of the difference is about the same throughout the last two-thirds of the study period.

10.5 Adaptive Spline Models   157

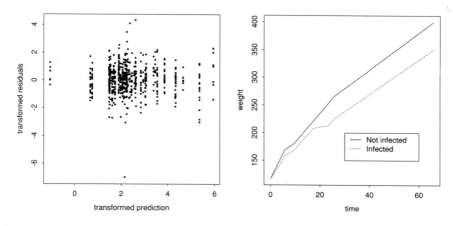

FIGURE 10.5. Residual plot (left) and the fitted growth curves (right).

To have a direct look into how well the model (10.30) fits the data, we plot the prediction curves together with the observations for infected and uninfected cows, respectively, in Figure 10.6. For the sake of comparison, the mean curves are also depicted in the figure. For the uninfected cows, the mean curve has more wiggle than the fitted curve, but otherwise they are close. For the infected cows, the fitted curve is practically identical to the mean curve. Therefore, it is evident from Figures 10.5 and 10.6 that model (10.30) provides a useful fit to the data.

Are the terms in the selected model (10.30) statistically significant? It is important to realize that MASAL selects models not based on the traditional standard of significance. Instead, it makes use of GCV. The two standards are clearly related, but generally they do not lead to the same model. In fact, because of the adaptive knot allocation and exhaustive search of basis functions, the GCV criterion is usually more stringent than the significance level of 0.05, as shown in Table 10.8. Assigning exact significance levels to the terms in (10.30) is an open question. Thus, we use a straightforward, but potentially biased, approach.

First, we hold the eight basis functions in (10.30) as if they were chosen prior to the model selection. Then, model (10.30) is a linear regression model. Table 10.8 shows the information related to the significance level of each term. All p-values are far below a traditional mark of 0.05.

In retrospect, all terms in model (10.30) are highly "significant" if we have certain faith in the p-values. Could iron dosing and the interaction between iron dosing and infection play a role that is nevertheless significant at a less ambitious level? To answer this question, we add x_2 and x_3, for example, to model (10.30). It turns out that x_2 and x_3 do not really affect the coefficients of the existing terms in model (10.30), and they are not significant at all (p-values > 0.5). This analysis confirms that of Diggle, Liang, and Zeger (1994). Interestingly, however, when fitting the

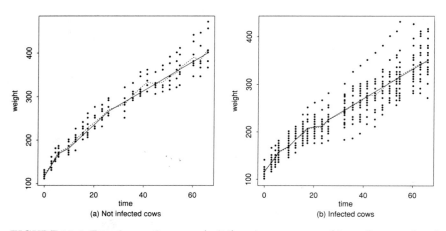

FIGURE 10.6. Fitted growth curves (solid) and mean curves (dotted) surrendered by the observed data points

TABLE 10.8. Significance of Model Parameters with Fixed Basis Functions

Basis function	t-Statistic	p-value
Intercept	47.5	$< 10^{-9}$
t	25.6	$< 10^{-9}$
$(t - 5.7)^+$	-11.8	$< 10^{-9}$
$(t - 9.7)^+$	6.1	$< 10^{-8}$
$(t - 25.8)^+$	-6.2	$< 10^{-8}$
tx_2	-5.0	$< 10^{-6}$
$(t - 4.4)^+ x_2$	4.0	0.00007
$(t - 17.4)^+ x_2$	-10.0	$< 10^{-9}$
$(t - 23.2)^+ x_2$	8.6	$< 10^{-9}$

log-weights, Zhang (1997) found that the interaction plays a significant role.

Example 10.3 *Blood Glucose Levels*

The data for this example are taken from Table 2.3 of Crowder and Hand (1990). Six students at Surrey University were offered free meals in exchange for having their blood glucose levels measured. Six test meals were given for each student at 10 a.m., 2 p.m., 6 a.m., 6 p.m., 2 a.m., and 10 p.m. Blood glucose levels were recorded ten times relatively to the meal time as follows. The first glucose level was measured 15 minutes before the meal, followed by a measurement at the meal time. The next four measurements were taken a half hour apart, and the last four (some five) measurements one hour apart. Figure 10.8 shows the growth curves of glucose level for different meal times with the first two records removed.

The primary issue is the time-of-day effect on the glucose variational pattern. Since the hours are periodic, we use x_1 to indicate the morning time and x_2 the afternoon time. Furthermore, we use three additional dummy variables, x_3 to x_5, to discriminate two meal times in each of the morning, afternoon, and night sessions. Because of the primary interest, we enter x_1 to x_5 into the model up front.

Crowder and Hand (1990, p. 13) conducted some preliminary analysis for these data, using the concept of the total area under the curve (AUC). In other words, if we take a subject at a meal time, we have a growth curve of glucose level. Above a reasonably chosen "basal" level there is an area under the curve. The information contributed by the curve is then compressed into a single number—the area. After this data compression, a simple t-test can be employed. The AUC is obviously an interpretable feature of the curve, whereas it contains limited information. Crowder and Hand also pointed out some fundamental limitations in the use of AUC. Here, we attempt to fit the glucose pattern as a function of meal time and measurement time. Furthermore, we will treat the first two measurements (before and at the meal time) as predictors instead of responses because they may reflect the up-to-date physical status of the subject.

As a prelude to the use of MASAL, we need to explore the covariance structure. As an initial attempt, we make use of the sample covariance matrix from the first-hand residuals that are obtained as follows. For every meal time and every measurement time, we have six glucose levels from the six students. It is easy to find the group average of these six levels. Then, the first-hand residuals are the glucose levels less their corresponding group averages. Using these residuals we plot in Figure 10.7 the sample variance against time (left) and the sample correlation against the lag (right). The figure also exhibits the estimated curves by the least squares method:

$$\hat{\sigma}^2(t) = \exp\left(0.535 - 0.0008t - 6.2t^2/10^5 + 1.4t^3/10^7\right) \qquad (10.31)$$

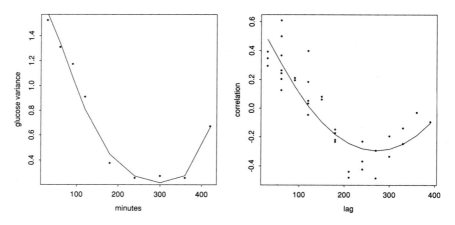

FIGURE 10.7. Initial covariance structure. The dots are the sample estimates and the curves the fitted values

and

$$\hat{\rho}(\Delta) = \sin\left(0.71 - 0.074\Delta + 1.4\Delta^2/10^5\right), \tag{10.32}$$

where t denotes time in minutes and Δ is the time lag. Note in (10.32) that we use a sinusoid function to ensure that the correlation is between -1 and 1, although the trend shows a roughly quadratic pattern.

We employ (10.31) and (10.32) to form the initial estimate of the covariance matrix. In the subsequent iterations, the covariance matrix will be estimated by the maximum likelihood method based on the residuals from the MASAL models.

We undertook three iterations for this example, and the changes from iteration to iteration were minor. In fact, the basis functions were nearly identical in the three iterations. There are changes in the estimates for the covariance parameters from the initial iteration to the second one, but little afterwards. The following MASAL model is from the third iteration:

$$8.5 - 0.5x_1 - 0.49x_2 - 0.017t + 0.016(t-220)^+, \tag{10.33}$$

led by the covariance structure

$$\hat{\sigma}^2(t) = \exp\left(1 - 0.0024t - 9.17t^2/10^5 + 1.87t^3/10^7\right)$$

and

$$\hat{\rho}(\Delta) = \sin\left(0.793 - 0.00857\Delta + 1.65\Delta^2/10^5\right).$$

From (10.33), we see that the glucose levels were higher when the test meals were given at night, but whether the meals were had in the morning or afternoon did not matter because the coefficients for x_1 and x_2 are very close. The glucose levels drops linearly for three and a half hours after the meal and then stays flat.

TABLE 10.9. Differences of Glucose Levels Between Different Meal Times

Dummy variables	Coefficient	S.E.	p-value
x_1	−0.46	0.142	0.001
x_2	−0.43	0.141	0.003
x_3	0.02	0.142	0.896
x_4	−0.03	0.147	0.863
x_5	0.10	0.135	0.447

Figure 10.8 compares the model (10.33) to the original paths of the glucose levels at 6 different meal times. Looking at the plots at the 10 a.m. meal time, the fit may not catch the underlying trend well enough. Some detailed features at the 10 p.m. meal time may be missed by the MASAL model. Overall, the MASAL model appears to reflect the underlying process of blood glucose levels.

After performing an AUC analysis, Crowder and Hand concluded that there was a significant difference of the glucose levels between 10 a.m. and 10 p.m. meals, which, in some aspects, is similar to what we stated above. Finally, we revert to the primary question, How different are the glucose levels at different meal times? To answer this, we use the old trick by adding x_3, x_4, and x_5 to model (10.33) at once. Table 10.9 reports the information for the five dummy variables only. The coefficients corresponding to x_3, x_4, and x_5 are practically inconsequential and statistically insignificant. Therefore, what seems to matter is whether the meals were given at night.

10.5.5 Analysis of Infant Growth Curves

In previous examples, we have used MASAL to fit the growth curve data that were collected with a relatively regular schedule. In Example 10.3, the blood glucose levels were measured at the same time for the six subjects. In many other situations such as the example in Section 10.1, data come from a rather irregular schedule due to various practical limitations. It is time for us to take a detailed look at the growth curves in presented in Section 10.1.

As opposed to the data in Examples 10.2 and 10.3, Figure 10.1 reveals a distinguished irregularity feature of the data: Different children made their visits during the study period at different ages (in days). This irregularity makes it difficult to scrutinize the covariance structure.

To assess the time trend for the variance at any time point d between 1 and 540 days, we collect a number of cross-sectional body weights, $\mathbf{z}_d$, from all children whose last visit was after d days. If a child visited the doctor on day d, the child's weight is included in $\mathbf{z}_d$. However, if a child visited the doctor before and after, but not on, day d, we include the interpolated value between the two adjacent weights in the shortest time interval containing

162   10. Analysis of Longitudinal Data

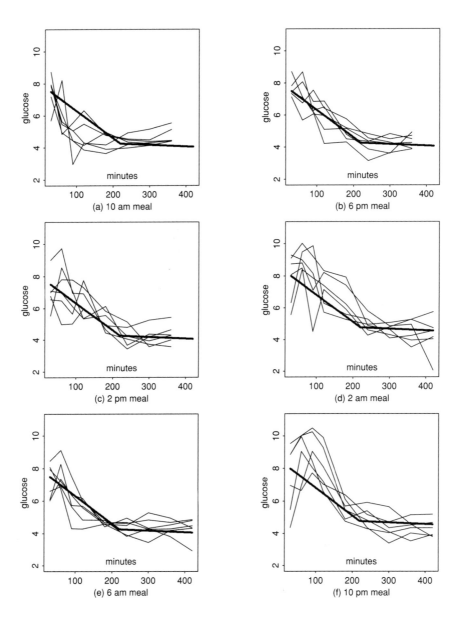

FIGURE 10.8. Blood glucose levels and the models. The thinner lines are individual paths, and the thicker ones the fits.

day d. This can be viewed as cutting the growth curves displayed in Figure 10.1 vertically on every day and then collecting all intersected points into z_d. Zhang (1999) found that the variance indeed increases with age and that the pattern can be adequately described by a cubic polynomial.

To fully specify the covariance structure, we also need to gauge the autocorrelation of weights between any two days. Because of the irregular time schedule, an efficient way of examining the autocorrelation is the use of the variogram (Diggle, Liang, and Zeger, 1994, pp. 50-51). For a stochastic process $Y(t)$, the variogram is defined as

$$\gamma(\Delta) = \frac{1}{2} E\{Y(t) - Y(t - \Delta)\}^2, \quad \Delta \geq 0.$$

If $Y(t)$ is stationary with variance σ^2, the autocorrelation is a simple transformation of the variogram as follows:

$$\rho(\Delta) = 1 - \gamma(\Delta)/\sigma^2.$$

Although we have realized that the variance is not constant over time, we hope that the variogram is still informative in revealing the autocorrelation structure.

To obtain the sample variogram as a function of lag, we proceeded in two steps following a procedure described by Diggle, Liang, and Zeger (1994, p. 51). First, we subtract each observation Y_{ij} on day d_{ij} from the average over a one-week period to derive an initial residual r_{ij}, $j = 1, \ldots, T_i$, $i = 1, \ldots, n$. Then, the sample variogram is calculated from pairs of half-squared residuals

$$v_{ijk} = \frac{1}{2}(r_{ij} - r_{ik})^2$$

with a lag of $\Delta_{ijk} = d_{ij} - d_{ik}$. At each value of lag Δ, the average of v is taken as the sample variogram $\hat{\gamma}(\Delta)$. Remarkably, Zhang (1999) discovered that the autocorrelation follows a linear trend.

After these explorations, it appears reasonable to postulate the following structure for the covariance structure:

$$\sigma^2(d) = \exp(\nu_0 + \nu_1 d + \nu_2 d^2 + \nu_3 d^3), \quad d = \text{day } 1, \ldots, \text{day } 540 \quad (10.34)$$

and

$$\rho(\Delta) = \phi_0 + \phi_1 \Delta, \quad \Delta = \text{lag } 1, \ldots, \text{lag } 539. \quad (10.35)$$

Model (10.1) results from using (10.34) and (10.35) as the backbone of the covariance matrix and going through the same iterative process as in the previous examples.

How well does the MASAL model fit the data? We address this question graphically. In Figure 10.9, we plot the residuals against the predicted values. In the original scale, as we expected, the variability is greater for a

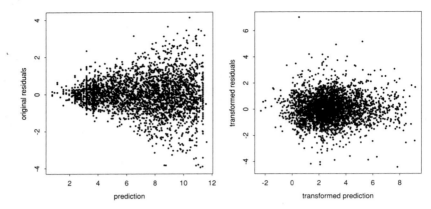

FIGURE 10.9. Residual plots against predictions (bottom). The left panel is in the original scale and the right one in a standardized scale.

larger predicted value (see the left panel). After transforming the residuals through the covariance matrix, no apparent structure emerges when the transformed residuals are plotted against the transformed prediction. Thus, these residual plots are in favor of the selected MASAL model and the covariance structure (10.34) and (10.35). To further evaluate the MASAL model, we plot the fitted curves surrendered by the observed points at gestational ages of 36 and 40 weeks and for boys and girls, respectively, in Figure 10.10. We chose 36 and 40 weeks because a 40-week delivery is a full-term pregnancy, and 36 weeks is one week short of a term delivery. It is clear that the fitted curves reside well in the midst of the observations although there remain unexplained variations. Therefore, it is evident from Figures 10.9 and 10.10 that the selected MASAL model is adequate and useful.

As we mentioned earlier, we are particularly interested in the effect of cocaine use by a pregnant woman on her child's growth. This variable, denoted by c previously, did not stand out in the MASAL model. This is clearly an indication of this factor's limited impact. We should also realize that our model-building and variable-selection procedures are not the same as the traditional ones. Could cocaine use contribute significantly to infant growth under a traditional sense? To answer this question, we use model (10.1) as our basis. Precisely, we hold all terms in this model as fixed and examine the contribution of c by including c as a main effect or an interaction term with one of the existing terms in addition to all terms already in model (10.1). Table 10.10 presents the significance of these individual terms, where the p-values are based on a two-sided t-test. Given the number of tests that were undertaken, two terms involving the interactions between cocaine use and gestational age may be worth pursuing. Overall,

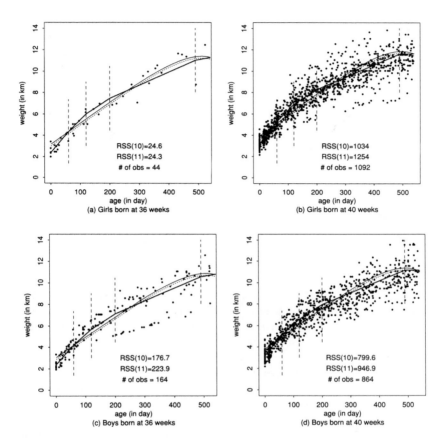

FIGURE 10.10. Observations and predictions for boys and girls born at 36 and 40 weeks. The thicker curves are from the MASAL model (10.1), and the vertical lines indicate the knot locations. Model (10.6) is drawn in thinner curves separately for the cocaine-use group (solid) and no-use group (dashed). Along with the number of observations, the unweighted residual sum of squares (RSS) is given respectively for models (10.1) and (10.6) inside each panel. This figure is reproduced from Figure 4 of Zhang (1999).

TABLE 10.10. The Impact of Cocaine Use on Infant Growth

Added term	Coefficient	t-statistic	p-value
c	0.162	2.42	0.016
cd	0.0004	1.37	0.17
$c(d-120)^+$	0.0003	0.96	0.34
$c(g_a-28)^+$	0.0166	2.69	0.007
$cd(g_a-28)^+$	0.00003	1.37	0.17
$c(d-60)^+(g_a-28)^+$	0.00005	1.68	0.093
$c(d-490+)^+(g_a-28)^+$	0.0001	0.35	0.73
csd	0.0002	1.10	0.27
$cs(d-120)^+$	0.0004	0.71	0.48
$c(d-200)^+$	0.0002	0.52	0.60

This table is reproduced from Zhang (1999)

our data do not support the hypothesis that cocaine use by a pregnant woman influences her infant's growth significantly.

10.5.6 Remarks

There are a number of research questions that are not explored here. The most important ones are whether the iterative procedure for estimating the covariance matrices converges, say, in probability, and how fast the convergence is. When no covariates but time are involved, our iterative procedure is analogous to the so-called iterated Cochrane–Orcutt procedure studied by Altman (1992). In one-dimensional smoothing with correlated errors, Truong (1991) and Altman (1992) provided some asymptotic and numerical properties for the covariance estimates after the first iteration. It would be interesting to extend their theoretical results to our iterative scheme. Truong (1991) assumed certain structures for the errors. It would be helpful to consider these structures when we apply MASAL for the analysis of longitudinal data.

Our examples have repeatedly shown that the MASAL model almost converges in the second iteration. This does not appear to be accidental, provided that the initial covariance matrix is constructed with "careful" thought. Next, we give a heuristic argument that supports the convergence of the iterative algorithm. This argument will also reveal where the convergence can be destroyed.

The convergence here refers to the gradual increase in the likelihood, l_r, defined in (10.22) as we move along with iterations. Suppose that we start with an initial covariance matrix Ψ_0, and f_0 is the resulting initial MASAL model. Then, the covariance matrix is reestimated by maximizing l_r while

f_0 is held fixed, giving Ψ_1. Clearly,

$$l_r(f_0, \Psi_1) = \max_{\Psi} l_r(f_0, \Psi) \geq l_r(f_0, \Psi_0). \tag{10.36}$$

Next, beginning at Ψ_1 we build another MASAL model, f_1, by minimizing the WSS defined in (10.12) or maximizing l_r for the given Ψ_1. If we indeed have

$$l_r(f_1, \Psi_1) = \max_{f \text{ in } (9.6)} \geq l_r(f_0, \Psi_1), \tag{10.37}$$

then $l_r(f_1, \Psi_1) \geq l_r(f_0, \Psi_0)$, which shows that l_r does not decrease from one iteration to the next. The relationship in (10.36) is granted if we assume a parametric covariance structure. Note critically, however, that MASAL does not really guarantee the expression (10.37) due to its stepwise nature. Moreover, the MASAL function f is chosen from a set of functions with infinite dimensions; thus, blindly maximizing l_r is not so meaningful, because larger models always have advantages over smaller ones. Note also that we have $l_r(f_1, \Psi_1) \geq l_r(f_0, \Psi_0)$ if $l_r(f_1, \Psi_1) \geq l_r(f_0, \Psi_1)$. If necessary, the MASAL algorithm can be modified to ensure the latter inequality. The key idea is to use f_0 as a reference while we build f_1, which is originally constructed from nothing. It warrants further investigation whether the step-by-step increase of l_r is at the price of missing a better model down the road.

10.6 Regression Trees for Longitudinal Data

Segal (1992) modified and used regression trees described in Section 9.9 to model longitudinal data. If continuity is not a major concern, regression trees provide a useful tool to stratify growth curves and help us answer questions such as, Do the growth curves of body weights of cows in Example 10.2 form covariate-specific clusters? MASAL does not explicitly extract meaningful subgroups of growth curves characterized by covariates, although it is straightforward to infer the subgroups from a MASAL model.

In theory, a regression tree model can be expressed by a function in (9.6), namely, a MARS model. In reality, tree-based methods and adaptive splines use different model-building techniques. As a consequence, they do not necessarily end up with the same model.

It is also important to clarify the applicability of the regression trees, as opposed to that of MASAL. We have seen that MASAL has no restriction on the data structure. In contrast, the regression trees as formulated by Segal (1992) can be applied to the longitudinal data with a regular structure. That is, all subjects should have the same number of observations and should be arranged for measurements at a well-defined, consistent schedule. A slight relaxation to this restriction will be discussed later.

In Section 9.9 we described regression trees in the ordinary regression setting. Again, we need a within-node impurity in tree growing and a cost-complexity criterion for tree pruning. So, we first establish the two key criteria and then expand our introduction by addressing other more technical issues.

For any node τ, let $\Psi(\boldsymbol{\theta}_\tau)$ be the within-node covariance matrix of the longitudinal responses and $\bar{\mathbf{y}}(\tau)$ the vector of within-node sample averages of the responses, where $\boldsymbol{\theta}_\tau$ is a vector of parameters that may depend on the node. Then, an obvious within-node impurity as measured by the least squares is

$$SS(\tau) = \sum_{\text{subject } i \in \tau} (\mathbf{y}_i - \bar{\mathbf{y}}(\tau))' \Psi^{-1}(\boldsymbol{\theta}_\tau)(\mathbf{y}_i - \bar{\mathbf{y}}(\tau)). \tag{10.38}$$

To split a node τ into its two daughter nodes, τ_L and τ_R, we aim at minimizing both $SS(\tau_L)$ and $SS(\tau_R)$. In other words, we maximize the split function

$$\phi(s, \tau) = SS(\tau) - SS(\tau_L) - SS(\tau_R), \tag{10.39}$$

where s is an allowable split. Moreover, it is also reasonable to define the tree cost as

$$R(\mathcal{T}) = \sum_{\tau \in \tilde{\mathcal{T}}} SS(\tau), \tag{10.40}$$

and then the cost-complexity (4.7) follows naturally.

To use (10.38) in the regression trees, we need to figure out the covariance matrix $\Psi(\boldsymbol{\theta}_\tau)$, as we did in MASAL. Conceptually, $\Psi(\boldsymbol{\theta}_\tau)$ is allowed to change from node to node. This relaxation can cause several problems, however. The split function, $\phi(s, \tau)$, is not guaranteed to be nonnegative. The cost of computation could be high. Most importantly, as the node size becomes smaller and smaller, it is more and more unrealistic to estimate the within-node covariance matrix precisely. Therefore, in practice, it is more likely than not that we would choose a pooled sample covariance structure for all nodes. Unlike MASAL, the regression trees of Segal (1992) do not iteratively update the covariance and tree structures.

As we pointed out earlier, the regression trees of Segal require a regular data structure. What can we do when the data are largely, but not perfectly, regular? Example 10.3 on the blood glucose levels is such a case, where there are a few missing responses, and one extra measurement was taken at three meal times between 10 p.m. and 6 a.m. Segal (1992) proposed to impute the missing responses using the EM algorithm (see, e.g., McLachlan and Krishnan, 1997). The merit of this solution is not clear. Some obvious concerns arise. The first one is the computational efficiency. More seriously, the imputation depends on the choice of the covariance structure. If the imputation procedure is not particularly sensitive to the misspecification of the covariance matrix, it is likely to produce reasonable and robust results. These issues are largely unexplored.

10.6.1 Example: HIV in San Francisco

In this section we illustrate regression trees with an application adapted from Segal (1992). We wish to express our special gratitude to Professor Mark Segal, at the University of California, San Francisco, who generously sent his postscript files for us to produce Figures 10.11–10.13.

In Chapter 7 we have highlighted the importance of estimating the incubation period from HIV infection to the onset of AIDS. The AIDS symptoms result from deterioration of the immune system. Thus, it is important to understand the natural history of this immune function decay in order to evaluate the therapeutic effects, to project the course of epidemic, etc.

The incubation period for AIDS is long (the median $\approx$ 10 years) and varies among individuals. This variability is hypothetically due to the existence of subgroups expressing distinct patterns of immune-function decay as measured by markers such as β_2 microglobulin. Segal (1992) utilized the regression trees to determine whether subgroups exist and, if so, whether these subgroups can be characterized in terms of covariates.

The analysis involves 96 subjects in a cohort of 462 homosexual men from sexually transmitted disease clinics, sexual partners of AIDS patients, and the San Francisco community from 1983 to 1984. Annual reports were made for the study participants with regard to information including sociodemographic, medical history, and immune markers. The 96 subjects were chosen because they had provided data on β_2 microglobulin for their first five annual visits, which consist of the response measurements. The covariates entered into the tree-based analysis include age; education; race; number of past episodes of syphilis, gonorrhea, genital herpes, and hepatitis B; number of male sex partners in the preceding year; history of blood transfusion; and smoking and alcohol consumption. All the covariates are baseline variables. Detailed study design has been described in Moss et al. (1988).

Based on the sample correlations, Segal used a compound symmetry covariance structure as defined in (10.17) and created the regression tree in Figure 10.11.

Figure 10.12 displays subgroup-specific individual curves of β_2 microglobulin corresponding to the nodes in Figure 10.11. The average profile of β_2 microglobulin for each node is shown in Figure 10.13.

From Figures 10.11–10.13, it appears that the less sexually active subjects, specifically those who had fewer than 28 male partners in the preceding year (node 2), had lower average levels of β_2 microglobulin than their more sexually active counterparts (node 3). Those more sexually active, but without past syphilis, subjects (node 4) had a similar average pro-

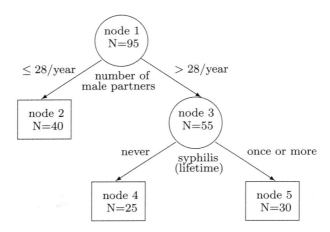

FIGURE 10.11. β_2 microglobulin regression tree. Adapted from Segal (1992).

file to those less sexually active subjects. The individuals who were more sexually active and had past syphilis had the worst immune-function loss. Further, Figure 10.13 also shows that the node-specific average profiles are not parallel. The rate of immune function loss for the subjects in node 3 is faster that that for the subjects in node 2, and likewise for nodes 4 and 5. It is noteworthy, however, that more sexually active individuals might have been infected earlier. In other words, the number of sex partners may not be the real cause, but instead it might have acted as a proxy for other important factors such as different infection times that were not available in the data.

10.6 Regression Trees for Longitudinal Data   171

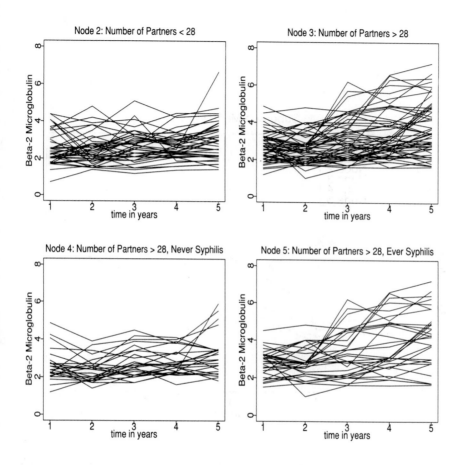

FIGURE 10.12. Patterns of β_2 microglobulin for all individuals in four nodes of the tree presented in Figure 10.11. This figure was composed using postscript files made by Mark Segal.

172   10. Analysis of Longitudinal Data

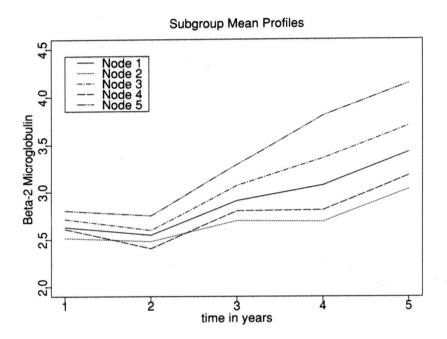

FIGURE 10.13. The average profile of β_2 microglobulin within each node of the tree presented in Figure 10.11. This figure was composed using a postscript file made by Mark Segal.

11
Analysis of Multiple Discrete Responses

In Chapter 10 we introduced some contemporary approaches to analyzing longitudinal data for which the responses are continuous measurements. In fact, most people imply continuous responses when they refer to longitudinal data. The analysis of discrete longitudinal data is a relatively new, though active, subject. Readers who are interested in methodological developments may find many unanswered questions in this chapter. The purpose of this chapter is to shed some light on this growing subject. In the statistical literature, the topic may be tagged with clustered or correlated discrete/binary outcomes. So far, most progress has been made toward the binary outcomes; hence, therein lies the focus of this chapter.

Sometimes, correlated discrete responses are generated from a single endpoint by repeatedly measuring it on individuals in a temporal or spatial domain. They are called longitudinal discrete responses. Examples 11.1 and 11.2 represent this class of data. Other times, as in Example 11.3 and in Section 11.3 the correlated responses consist of distinct endpoints. In recent years, we have witnessed more and more studies that involve both types of responses, such as Example 11.4.

Example 11.1 To investigate racial differences in the cause-specific prevalence of blindness, Sommer et al. (1991) used a randomly selected, stratified, multistage cluster sample of 2,395 Blacks and 2,913 Whites 40 years of age and older in East Baltimore. Those 5,208 subjects underwent detailed ophthalmic examinations by a single team. In this study, the authors observed bivariate binary responses in a spatial domain for each subject, namely, the blindness of left and right eyes. The authors found that the leading causes of blindness were unoperated senile cataract, primary open-angle glaucoma, and age-related macular degeneration. They also concluded that the pattern of blindness in urban Baltimore appears to be different among Blacks and Whites. Whites are far more likely to have age-related macular degeneration, and Blacks to have primary open-angle glaucoma. Subsequently, Liang, Zeger, and Qaqish (1992) reanalyzed these data, comparing different statistical approaches.

Example 11.2 From 1974 to 1977, a team of investigators conducted a longitudinal study of the respiratory health effects of air pollutants among children and adults living in six cities in the United States. The study design was reported by Ferris et al. (1979) and Sommer et al. (1984). The selection of the cities was to cover a range of air quality based on their historic levels of outdoor pollution. In all but one small city, the initial examinations included all first- and second-grade school children. In the small city, children up to the fifth grade were included. The study subjects were reexamined annually for three years. At each visit, the investigators collected information regarding the number of persons living in the house, familial smoking habits, parental occupation and education background, the fuel used for cooking in the house, pulmonary function, respiratory illness history, and symptom history. In Ware et al. (1984), they selected 10,106 children 6 to 9 years of age at the enrollment and analyzed wheeze status (yes, no) of the children as a longitudinal binary outcome. Additional analyses have been conducted by Zeger, Liang, and Albert (1988) and Fitzmaurice and Laird (1993) among others.

Example 11.3 This is an example where the risk of two distinct, but presumably correlated, outcomes were studied, i.e., respiratory disease and diarrhea in children with preexisting mild vitamin A deficiency.

Sommer and colleagues (Sommer et al., 1983 and 1984) conducted a prospective longitudinal study of 4,600 children aged up to 6 years at entry in rural villages of Indonesia between March 1977 and December 1978. Their research team examined these children every 3 months for 18 months. An average of 3,135 children were free of respiratory disease and diarrhea at the examination. At each examination, they recorded interval medical history, weight, height, general health status, and eye condition. They found that the risk of respiratory disease and diarrhea were more closely associated with vitamin A status than with general nutritional status.

Example 11.4 Genes underlie numerous conditions and diseases. A vast number of genetic epidemiologic studies have been conducted to infer genetic bases of various syndromes. Multiple clustered responses naturally arise from such studies. For example, Scourfield et al. (1996) examined the gender difference in disorders of substance abuse, comorbidity anxiety, and sensation seeking, using the database from the Genetic Epidemiology Research Unit, Yale University School of Medicine, New Haven, Connecticut,

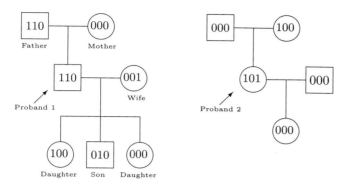

FIGURE 11.1. Two pedigrees of different family sizes. Each square or circle represents a family member. The left pedigree pinpoints the relationship of relatives to the proband. A sequence of three bits (0 or 1) is displayed within all squares and circles, marking the status of substance abuse, anxiety, and sensation seeking, respectively.

under the leadership of Professor Kathleen Merikangas. Two hundred sixty-two probands, through whom the other family members are ascertained, are included in the database. Information regarding a variety of psychiatric disorders and predictive covariates, e.g., gender, has been recorded for all probands and some of their relatives (parents, siblings, offspring, etc.). The pedigrees in Figure 11.1 illustrate typical family structures. We should note that the first proband has six relatives in the record, whereas the second one has four. In other words, the family size varies from pedigree to pedigree. It is also important to realize that multiple disorders, i.e., three, are evaluated for every member of a family.

11.1 Parametric Methods for Binary Responses

Suppose that $\mathbf{Y}_i = (Y_{i1}, \ldots, Y_{iq_i})'$ is a vector of binary responses for subject i, $i = 1, \ldots, n$. In Example 11.1, $q_i = 2$ for all 2,913 subjects, and (Y_1, Y_2) indicates the blindness of the left and right eyes. Likewise, we can easily define the response vector for Examples 11.2 and 11.3.

Parametric models have dominated the applications involving multiple binary responses. Log-linear and marginal models are in the spotlight in the literature. We give a brief discussion of these two models and strongly recommend reading related articles and books cited in this chapter.

11.1.1 Log-Linear Models

One of the most popular and conceptually simple models for multiple binary responses is the log-linear model that assumes the joint probability of $\mathbf{Y}_i$ to be of the form

$$I\!\!P\{\mathbf{Y}_i = \mathbf{y}_i\} = \exp\left[\sum_{j=1}^{q_i} \theta_{ij} y_{ij} + \sum_{j_1 < j_2} \theta_{ij_1 j_2} y_{ij_1} y_{ij_2} + \cdots \right.$$
$$\left. + \theta_{i1\cdots q_i} y_{i1} \cdots y_{iq_i} + A_i(\boldsymbol{\theta}_i)\right], \quad (11.1)$$

where

$$\boldsymbol{\theta}_i = (\theta_{i1}, \ldots, \theta_{iq_i}, \theta_{i12} \ldots \theta_{i,q_i-1,q_i}, \ldots, \theta_{1\cdots q_i})$$

is the $(2^{q_i-1} - 1)$-vector of canonical parameters and $\exp[A_i(\boldsymbol{\theta}_i)]$ is the normalizing constant.

Model (11.1) appears to involve too many parameters. In practice, however, it is usually greatly simplified. Two steps are critical to this simplification. First, most data are regular in the sense that the components of $\boldsymbol{\theta}_i$ correspond to fixed coordinates. In other words, $\boldsymbol{\theta}_i$ does not depend on i, and this subscript can be removed. In Examples 11.1–11.3, the vector of canonical parameters, $\boldsymbol{\theta}_i$, does not depend on i. For instance, Example 11.3 involves only $2^2 - 1 = 3$ parameters. Second, the canonical parameters with respect to the terms with the third- or higher-orders are generally hypothetically set to zero. The resulting models are referred to as the quadratic exponential model (see, e.g., Zhao and Prentice, 1990; Fitzmaurice and Laird, 1995). Estimating those "removed" parameters could otherwise raise a tremendous challenge to data analysis.

In family studies as illustrated by Example 11.4, the vector of canonical parameters, $\boldsymbol{\theta}_i$, may not have a fixed coordinate system. Although the number of interested disorders is three for every subject, the size of pedigree differs when the entire pedigree is regarded as a unit, or cluster. In such applications, it is vital to form a parametric system that reflects the nature of $\mathbf{Y}_i$. This practice depends, however, on individual applications.

Next, let us take a look at the quadratic exponential model in which the canonical parameters have a fixed coordinate system:

$$I\!\!P\{\mathbf{Y} = \mathbf{y}\} = \exp\left[\sum_{j=1}^{q} \theta_j y_j + \sum_{j<k} \theta_{jk} y_j y_k + A(\boldsymbol{\theta})\right], \quad (11.2)$$

where

$$\boldsymbol{\theta} = (\theta_1, \ldots, \theta_q, \theta_{12} \cdots \theta_{q-1,q}).$$

Based on model (11.2), the canonical parameters have certain interpretations. Precisely, we have

$$\log\left[\frac{I\!\!P\{Y_j = 1 | Y_k = y_k, Y_l = 0, l \neq j, k\}}{I\!\!P\{Y_j = 0 | Y_k = y_k, Y_l = 0, l \neq j, k\}}\right] = \theta_j + \theta_{jk} y_k.$$

11.1 Parametric Methods for Binary Responses

Thus, θ_j is the log odds for $Y_j = 1$ given that the remaining components of Y equal zero. In addition, θ_{jk} is referred to as an association parameter because it is the conditional log odds ratio describing the association between Y_j and Y_k provided that the other components of Y are zero. It is important to realize that the canonical parameters are the log odds or odds ratio under certain conditions, but we should be aware of the fact that these conditions may not always make sense.

Why is model (11.1) called a log-linear model? Let us consider a bivariate case. It follows from model (11.2) that the joint probability for the n bivariate vectors is

$$\exp[\theta_1(n_{21} + n_{22}) + \theta_2(n_{12} + n_{22}) + \theta_{12}n_{22} + nA(\boldsymbol{\theta})], \tag{11.3}$$

where $n_{11} = \sum_{i=1}^{n}(1-y_{i1})(1-y_{i2})$, $n_{12} = \sum_{i=1}^{n}(1-y_{i1})y_{i2}$, $n_{21} = \sum_{i=1}^{n} y_{i1}(1-y_{i2})$, and $n_{22} = \sum_{i=1}^{n} y_{i1}y_{i2}$ are the cell counts in the following 2 × 2 table:

		Y_2	
		0	1
Y_1	0	n_{11}	n_{12}
	1	n_{21}	n_{22}

It is easy to see that the expression in (11.3) equals

$$\frac{n!}{n_{11}!n_{12}!n_{21}!n_{22}!} m_{11}^{n_{11}} m_{12}^{n_{12}} m_{21}^{n_{21}} m_{22}^{n_{22}},$$

where

$$\log(m_{jk}) = \mu + \lambda_j^{Y_1} + \lambda_k^{Y_2} + \lambda_{jk}^{Y_1Y_2}, \tag{11.4}$$

with

$$\mu = (\theta_1 + \theta_2)/2 + \theta_{12}/4 + A(\boldsymbol{\theta}), \tag{11.5}$$
$$\lambda_1^{Y_1} = -\theta_1/2 - \theta_{12}/4 + A(\boldsymbol{\theta}), \tag{11.6}$$
$$\lambda_1^{Y_2} = -\theta_2/2 - \theta_{12}/4 + A(\boldsymbol{\theta}), \tag{11.7}$$
$$\lambda_{11}^{Y_1Y_2} = \theta_{12}/4, \tag{11.8}$$

and $\lambda_2^{Y_1} = -\lambda_1^{Y_1}$, $\lambda_2^{Y_2} = -\lambda_1^{Y_2}$, and $\lambda_{12}^{Y_1Y_2} = \lambda_{21}^{Y_1Y_2} = -\lambda_{22}^{Y_1Y_2} = -\lambda_{11}^{Y_1Y_2}$. In other words, $(n_{11}, n_{12}, n_{21}, n_{22})$ follows a multinomial distribution with means specified by the log-linear effects in (11.4). This is usually how the log-linear models are introduced (e.g., Agresti, 1990, Chapter 5). Further, equations (11.5)–(11.8) provide another way to interpret the canonical parameters.

11.1.2 Marginal Models

As we mentioned earlier, the interpretation of canonical parameters in the log-linear model depends on certain conditions that are not always of clinical relevance. On the other hand, after the reformation of the log-linear model in (11.4), the canonical parameters have one-to-one relationships with the "marginal" parameters as delineated in (11.5)–(11.8). Here, the marginal parameters refer to the main and interactive effects in model (11.4). For many investigators, the question of utmost importance is related to the marginal parameters that are defined directly from the marginal distribution of the responses, unlike the canonical parameters, which involve all responses at once.

One possibility is to reparameterize the log-linear model in terms of marginal means, correlations, etc. In fact, the Bahadur representation is another typical method to represent the log-linear model, and it directly extends the multinomial distribution by including additional multiplicative factors to take into account the association among the components of $\mathbf{Y}$ (Bahadur 1961; Fitzmaurice et al., 1993; Diggle et al., 1994). In mathematical form, we have

$$P\{\mathbf{Y} = \mathbf{y}\} = \prod_{j=1}^{q} \mu_j^{y_j}(1-\mu_j)^{(1-y_j)}$$
$$\times (1 + \sum_{j_1<j_2} \rho_{j_1 j_2} r_{j_1} r_{j_2} + \sum_{j_1<j_2<j_3} \rho_{j_1 j_2 j_3} r_{j_1} r_{j_2} r_{j_3} + \cdots + \rho_{1 \cdots q} r_1 \cdots r_q),$$

where

$$\mu_j = E\{Y_j\},$$
$$r_j = (y_j - \mu_j)/\sqrt{\mu_j(1-\mu_j)},$$
$$\rho_{j_1 \cdots j_l} = E\{R_{j_1} \cdots R_{j_l}\},$$

$j = 1, \ldots, q$.

The Bahadur representation is one step forward in terms of formulating the log-linear model as a function of the parameters such as means and correlations that we used to see in the analysis of continuous responses. This representation is, however, severely handicapped by the fact that the "hierarchal" correlations entangle the ones at lower-orders and the means and that it is particularly problematic in the presence of covariates. To address the dilemma between the parameter interpretability and feasibility, Liang et al. (1992) proposed the use of marginal models parameterized by the means, the odds ratios, and the contrasts of odds ratios. Specifically,

let
$$\gamma_{j_1 j_2} = OR(Y_{j_1}, Y_{j_2}) = \frac{I\!P\{Y_{j_1}=1, Y_{j_2}=1\} I\!P\{Y_{j_1}=0, Y_{j_2}=0\}}{I\!P\{Y_{j_1}=1, Y_{j_2}=0\} I\!P\{Y_{j_1}=0, Y_{j_2}=1\}},$$
$$\zeta_{j_1 j_2 j_3} = \log[OR(Y_{j_1}, Y_{j_2}|Y_{j_3}=1)] - \log[OR(Y_{j_1}, Y_{j_2}|Y_{j_3}=0)],$$

and generally,

$$\zeta_{j_1 \cdots j_l} = \sum_{y_{j_3},\ldots,y_{j_l}=0,1} (-1)^{b(\mathbf{y})} \log[OR(Y_{j_1}, Y_{j_2}|y_{j_3},\ldots,y_{j_l})],$$

where $b(\mathbf{y}) = \sum_{k=3}^{l} y_{j_k} + l - 2$.

It is quite unfortunate that evaluating the full likelihood based on the new set of parameters, μ_j, $\gamma_{j_1 j_2}$, and $\zeta_{j_1 \cdots j_l}$, is generally complicated. To gain insight into where the complications arise, let us go through the details for the bivariate case. We need to specify the probability $I\!P\{Y_1 = y_1, Y_2 = y_2\} \stackrel{def}{=} p(y_1, y_2)$ for four possible combinations of (y_1, y_2). The following four equations can lead to the unique identification of the four probabilities:

$$\begin{aligned} p(1,1) + p(1,0) &= \mu_1, \\ p(0,1) + p(1,1) &= \mu_2, \\ p(1,1) + p(1,0) + p(0,1) + p(0,0) &= 1, \\ p(1,1)p(0,0) &= \gamma_{12} p(0,1) p(1,0). \end{aligned}$$

From the first three equations, we have $p(1,0) = \mu_1 - p(1,1)$, $p(0,1) = \mu_2 - p(1,1)$, and $p(0,0) = 1 - \mu_1 - \mu_2 + p(1,1)$. If we plug them into the last equation, we have a quadratic equation in $p(1,1)$,

$$(1-\gamma_{12})p^2(1,1) + [1 + (\gamma_{12}-1)(\mu_1+\mu_2)]p(1,1) - \gamma_{12}\mu_1\mu_2 = 0,$$

and the solution for $p(1,1) \stackrel{def}{=} \mu_{11}$ is (Dale, 1986)

$$\begin{cases} \frac{1+(\gamma_{12}-1)(\mu_1+\mu_2)-\{[1+(\gamma_{12}-1)(\mu_1+\mu_2)]^2+4(1-\gamma_{12})\gamma_{12}\mu_1\mu_2\}^{-\frac{1}{2}}}{2(1-\gamma_{12})} & \text{if } \gamma_{12} \neq 1, \\ \mu_1 \mu_2 & \text{if } \gamma_{12} = 1. \end{cases}$$

Using this solution, it is easy to conclude that

$$p(y_1, y_2) = \mu_1^{y_1}(1-\mu_1)^{1-y_1} \mu_2(1-\mu_2)^{1-y_2} + (-1)^{y_1-y_2}(\mu_{11} - \mu_1\mu_2).$$

When we have more than two responses, the problem could be intractable if we do not reduce the dimension of the parameters appropriately such as setting $\gamma_{j_1 j_2} = \gamma$.

11.1.3 Parameter Estimation*

In the log-linear and marginal models we have not introduced covariates. As a matter of fact, the question of most interest to us is to model the

180   11. Analysis of Multiple Discrete Responses

distribution of **Y** in the presence of covariates as in the previous chapters. In principle, it is straightforward to incorporate a set of the covariates, **x**, into the models. The canonical parameters $\boldsymbol{\theta}$ in the log-linear model (11.2) and the marginal parameters in the marginal models can be defined as a function of **x**, which is called the link function in the context of generalized linear models (McCullagh and Nelder, 1991, p. 27).

Depending on the specification of the link function, finding the maximum likelihood estimates of the parameters is not impossible; see, e.g., Section 11.2.3. Nevertheless, a more common practice is to make use of so-called generalized estimating equations (GEE), which simplify the estimation process while retaining some of the most important asymptotic properties of the estimates as elaborated below (Liang and Zeger, 1986).

Now, let us turn back to model (11.2) and explain how to use the idea of generalized estimating equations. First, we reexpress the probability in vector form:

$$\mathbb{P}\{\mathbf{Y} = \mathbf{y}\} = \exp[\boldsymbol{\theta}'\mathbf{z} - A(\boldsymbol{\theta})], \qquad (11.9)$$

where $\mathbf{z} = (\mathbf{y}', \mathbf{w}')'$ and **w** is a $\binom{q}{2}$-vector consisting of $(y_1 y_2, \ldots, y_{q-1} y_q)'$.

For model (11.9), we assume that there exists a vectorial link function $\boldsymbol{\eta}$ that transforms **x** coupled with a condensed vector of parameters $\boldsymbol{\beta}$ to $\boldsymbol{\theta}$, e.g., $\boldsymbol{\theta} = \boldsymbol{\eta}(\mathbf{x}'\boldsymbol{\beta})$. Then, the GEE approach attempts to solve the unbiased estimating equations (Godambe, 1960; Zhao and Prentice, 1990)

$$U(\boldsymbol{\beta}) = \sum_{i=1}^{n} JV_i^{-1} \begin{pmatrix} \mathbf{y}_i - \boldsymbol{\mu} \\ \mathbf{w}_i - \boldsymbol{\omega} \end{pmatrix} = 0, \qquad (11.10)$$

where $\boldsymbol{\omega} = \mathbb{E}\{\mathbf{w}\}$, $V_i = \text{Cov}(\mathbf{z}_i)$, and $J = \partial \boldsymbol{\theta}/\partial \boldsymbol{\beta}'$.

Liang et al. (1992) called (11.10) GEE2, because it is a second-order extension of the estimating equations proposed by Liang and Zeger (1986). However, if we set the block off-diagonal matrices in J and V_i to zero in (11.10), then (11.10) becomes GEE1, which can be less efficient than GEE2 when the link function is misspecified. We should also note that the block off-diagonal elements of the covariance matrix V_i cannot be determined by $\boldsymbol{\mu}$ and $\boldsymbol{\omega}$. To avoid estimating additional parameters, so-called working matrices are usually used to replace the underlying matrices (Zhao and Prentice, 1990).

The solution $\hat{\boldsymbol{\beta}}$ to (11.10) has, asymptotically as $n \to \infty$, a multivariate normal distribution with mean 0 and covariance matrix that can be consistently estimated by

$$\left(\sum_{i=1}^{n} JV_i J'\right)^{-1} \left(\sum_{i=1}^{n} JV_i \begin{pmatrix} \mathbf{y}_i - \boldsymbol{\mu} \\ \mathbf{w}_i - \boldsymbol{\omega} \end{pmatrix} \begin{pmatrix} \mathbf{y}_i - \boldsymbol{\mu} \\ \mathbf{w}_i - \boldsymbol{\omega} \end{pmatrix}' V_i J'\right) \left(\sum_{i=1}^{n} JV_i J'\right)^{-1}$$

evaluated at $\hat{\boldsymbol{\beta}}$ (Liang et al., 1992). It also turns that $U(\boldsymbol{\beta})$ resembles the quasi-score function derived from the quasi-likelihood as introduced in (9.5) of McCullagh and Nelder (1991).

Likewise, if we are interested in the pairwise odds ratio and use the marginal models, then we assume a link function between parameters μ_j and γ_{jk}, and covariates $\mathbf{x}$. The rest of the derivation for GEE is identical to that above.

11.1.4 Frailty Models

In Example 11.4, we have encountered different numbers of binary responses among different measurement units, namely families. Let the data for family i consist of binary responses Y_{ij} and covariates $\mathbf{x}_{ij}$, $j = 1, 2, \ldots, n_i$, $i = 1, 2, \ldots, I$. Here, I is the number of families, and n_i is the number of relatives in the ith family, $i = 1, 2, \ldots, I$.

In such family studies, the association of the health condition between relatives is of interest. One approach is to generalize the log-linear model introduced in Section 11.1.1 and to include higher-order interaction terms. Particularly, based on Connolly and Liang (1988), we may assume

$$\text{logit} I\!\!P\{Y_{ij} = 1 | Y_{il}, l \neq j, \mathbf{x}_i\} = F_{n_i}(W_{ij}; \theta) + \mathbf{x}_{ij}\boldsymbol{\beta}, \tag{11.11}$$

where $W_{ij} = \sum_{l \neq j}^{n_i} Y_{il}$, F_{n_i} is an arbitrary function, and θ is a parameter. This leads to the joint probability for the outcome in the ith family

$$\log I\!\!P\{\mathbf{Y}_i = \mathbf{y}_i | \mathbf{x}_i\} = \alpha + \sum_{j=1}^{n_i} y_{ij}\mathbf{x}_{ij}\boldsymbol{\beta} + \sum_{l=0}^{W_i + y_{ij} - 1} F_{n_i}(l; \theta). \tag{11.12}$$

Related to model (11.12), Bonney (1986, 1987) introduced several classes of regressive logistic models, assuming simple Markovian structures of dependence among the traits of family members. In essence, these regressive logistic models are ordinary logistic regression models except that the "covariates" are derived from a set of common-sense covariates and the outcomes of other family members. The regressive logistic models are practically appealing and have been widely used in segregation analysis.

Babiker and Cuzick (1994) noted two major problems with model (11.12) and its like. First, the parameterization depends on the family size n_i, and the coefficients obtained from different families are irreconcilable. Second, they pointed out that the conditional coefficients often are not easily converted to parameters of interest even when the family sizes are the same. For these concerns, they proposed the use of a simple frailty model. In most family studies, however, their simple one-frailty model cannot address questions of importance. To this end, it is useful to enhance the simple frailty model by considering the relationship among relatives.

Let us take the three-generation pedigree in Figure 11.1 as an example. We can introduce three types of unobserved frailties U_1^i, U_2^i, and U_3^i for the

ith family that represent common, unmeasured environmental factors; genetic susceptibility of the family founders; and the transmission of relevant genetic materials from a parent to a child. Here, a family founder is an individual whose parents were not sampled in the pedigree. To avoid technical complications, suppose that these frailties are independent Bernoulli random variables; that is,

$$I\!P\{U_k^i = 1\} = \theta_k = 1 - I\!P\{U_k^i = 0\},$$

for $k = 1, 2, 3$. A critical assumption is that for the ith family and conditional on all possible U_k^i's, denoted by U^i, the health conditions of all family members are independent and

$$\text{logit}(I\!P\{Y_j^i = 1|U^i\}) = \mathbf{x}_j^i \boldsymbol{\beta} + \mathbf{a}_j^i \boldsymbol{\gamma}, \qquad (11.13)$$

where $\boldsymbol{\beta}$ and $\boldsymbol{\gamma}$ are vectors of parameters, and

$$\mathbf{a}_j^i = (U_1^i, U_{2,2j-1}^i + U_{2,2j}^i, U_{2,2j-1}^i U_{2,2j}^i)'$$

harbors the frailties. The construction of $\mathbf{a}_j^i$ is based on assuming the existence of a major susceptibility locus with alleles A and a, as clarified below.

The frequency of allele A is θ_2, and $(U_{2,2j-1}^i, U_{2,2j}^i)$ indicate the presence of allele A in the two chromosomes of the jth member of the ith family. Based on the Mendelian transmission, $\theta_3 = 0.5$. The parameter interpretation in model (11.13) is most important. The β parameters measure the strength of association between the trait and the covariates conditional on the frailties, while the γ parameters indicate the familial and genetic contributions to the trait. Note that $\boldsymbol{\gamma} = (\gamma_1, \gamma_2, \gamma_3)'$. If $\gamma_2 = 0$ and $\gamma_3 \neq 0$, it suggests a recessive trait because a genetic effect is expressed only in the presence of two A alleles. On the other hand, if a completely dominant gene underlie the trait, genotypes Aa and AA give rise to the same effect, implying that $\gamma_2 = 2\gamma_2 + \gamma_3$, i.e., $\gamma_2- = \gamma_3$.

The frailty model (11.13) is closely related to many existing models for segregation analysis, all of which can be traced back to the classic Elston-Stewart (1971) model for the genetic analysis of pedigree data. The Elston-Stewart model was originally designed to identify the mode of inheritance of a particular trait of interest without considering the presence of covariates. The frailty model (11.13) is quite similar to the class D logistic regressive models of Bonney (1986, 1987). The major difference is the method for modeling familial correlations as a result of residual genetic effects and environment. The regressive models make use of the parental traits and assume the conditional independence among siblings on the parental traits. In contrast, the frailty model assumes the conditional independence among all family members on the frailty variable. Conceptually, frailty variables defined here are very similar to that of ousiotype introduced by Cannings et al. (1978) in pedigree analysis, where a unique ousiotype (essence) for each individual is assumed to represent unobservable genetic effects. Many other authors including Bonney (1986, 1987) adopted the ousiotype as the genotype. Frailty model (11.13) can be viewed as a further clarification of the ousiotype into a major genotype of focus and residual unobservable effects.

In terms of computation, when both U and Y are observable, the complete log-likelihood function is easy to derive, and the EM algorithm (Dempster, Laird, and Rubin, 1977) can be applied to find the parameter estimates. A detailed development of the frailty model for segregation analysis will be presented elsewhere (Zhang and Merikangas, 1999).

11.2 Classification Trees for Multiple Binary Responses

Many applications of parametric models have a notable common feature. That is, the models usually involve relatively few covariates, and there is little discussion of model selection. Although the theoretical models are not confined by the number of covariates, the reality of specifying parametric candidate models and then selecting the final model can be a serious challenge. To resolve this practical problem, Zhang (1998a) considered various automated approaches under the tree paradigm as a complement to the existing parametric methods. The discussions here are based on the work of Zhang (1998a).

11.2.1 Within-Node Homogeneity

Without exception, we need to define a new splitting function and cost-complexity in order to extend classification trees for the analysis of multiple discrete responses. First, we show how to generalize the entropy criterion (4.3) to the present situation making use of the log-linear model (11.9). We use the same idea as we derived (2.1). For the sake of simplicity, we assume that the joint distribution of $\mathbf{Y}$ depends on the linear terms and the sum of the second-order products of its components only. That is, we assume that the joint probability distribution of $\mathbf{Y}$ is

$$f(\mathbf{y}; \Psi, \theta) = \exp(\Psi'\mathbf{y} + \theta w - A(\Psi, \theta)), \quad (11.14)$$

where $w = \sum_{i<j} y_i y_j$. Now we define the generalized entropy criterion, or the homogeneity of node τ_L, as the maximum of the log-likelihood derived from this distribution, which equals

$$h(\tau_L) = \sum_{\{\text{subject } i \in \tau_L\}} (\hat{\Psi}'\mathbf{y}_i + \hat{\theta} w_i - A(\hat{\Psi}, \hat{\theta})), \quad (11.15)$$

where $\hat{\Psi}$ and $\hat{\theta}$ may be viewed as the maximum likelihood estimates of Ψ and θ, respectively. Obviously, the homogeneity of node t_R can be defined by analogy. The node impurity $i(\tau)$ can be chosen as $-h(\tau)$ if you will. Having defined the homogeneity (or impurity) measure, we plug it into (2.3) to form a splitting rule.

In addition to the homogeneity (11.15), there are other possibilities worth considering. If the responses were continuous, it would be natural to measure the node homogeneity through their covariance matrix. Therefore, it is reasonable to explore a homogeneity measure via a covariance matrix such as (10.38) for regression trees.

Within a node τ, we can measure its homogeneity (counter variation) in terms of the distribution of $\mathbf{Y}$ by

$$h_1(\tau) = -\log |V_\tau|, \tag{11.16}$$

where $|V_\tau|$ is the determinant of the within-node sample covariance matrix of $\mathbf{Y}$. The use of the logarithm is to ensure the subadditivity

$$n_\tau h_1(\tau) \leq n_{\tau_L} h_1(\tau_L) + n_{\tau_R} h_1(\tau_R),$$

where n_τ, n_{τ_L}, and n_{τ_R} are respectively the numbers of subjects in node τ and its left and right daughter nodes τ_L and τ_R.

When we have a single binary response, criterion (11.16) is essentially the Gini index in (4.4). This is because

$$|V_\tau| = \frac{n_\tau}{n_\tau - 1} p_\tau (1 - p_\tau),$$

where p_τ is the proportion of diseased subjects in node τ.

Further, as a direct extension from the criterion (10.38) used in the trees for continuous longitudinal data, another measure of within-node homogeneity that deserves our attention is

$$h_2(\tau) = -\frac{1}{n_\tau} \sum_{i \in \text{node } \tau} (\mathbf{y}_i - \bar{\mathbf{y}}(\tau))' V^{-1} (\mathbf{y}_i - \bar{\mathbf{y}}(\tau)), \tag{11.17}$$

where V^{-1} is the covariance matrix of $\mathbf{Y}_i$ in the root node.

Finally, based on the discussion in the previous section, it would be more appropriate to replace the covariance matrix V_τ with a matrix constituted by the pairwise odds ratios when we deal with multiple binary responses. The consequence warrants further investigation.

11.2.2 Terminal Nodes

To construct a useful tree structure, a rigorous rule is warranted to determine the terminal nodes and hence the size of the tree. As in Section 4.2.2, we need to prepare a tree cost-complexity,

$$R_\alpha(\mathcal{T}) = R(\mathcal{T}) + \alpha |\tilde{\mathcal{T}}|,$$

11.2 Classification Trees for Multiple Binary Responses

as was first introduced in (4.7). Zhang (1998a) considered three definitions for the cost $R(\mathcal{T})$ with respect to h, h_1, and h_2. Using $h(\tau)$ he defined

$$R(\mathcal{T}) = -\sum_{\tau \in \tilde{\mathcal{T}}} \sum_{\{\text{subject } i \in \tau\}} \log f(\mathbf{y}_i; \hat{\Psi}, \hat{\theta}), \qquad (11.18)$$

where f is introduced in (11.14), and $\hat{\Psi}$ and $\hat{\theta}$ are estimated from the learning sample. Note, however, that subject i may or may not be included in the learning sample.

Using $h_1(\tau)$ Zhang introduced

$$R_1(\mathcal{T}) = -\sum_{\tau \in \tilde{\mathcal{T}}} n_\tau \log |V_\tau|,$$

where V_τ is the covariance matrix of $\mathbf{Y}$ within node τ with the average obtained from the learning sample even though $\mathbf{Y}$ may not be included in the learning sample. It turned out that $h_1(\tau)$ and $R_1(\mathcal{T})$ are not as useful as the other choices. For the data in Section 11.3, $h_1(\tau)$ in (11.16) suffered an undesirable end-cut preference problem. This phenomenon was described at the end of Section 2.2 as a side effect of using the Gini index for a single binary outcome. Because $h_1(\tau)$ can be viewed as a generalization of the Gini index, it is not surprising that $h_1(\tau)$ manifested the problem. Thus, we remove $h_1(\tau)$ and $R_1(\mathcal{T})$ from further discussion.

Likewise, for $h_2(\tau)$ we have

$$R_2(\mathcal{T}) = -\sum_{\tau \in \tilde{\mathcal{T}}} \sum_{\{\text{subject } i \in \tau\}} (\mathbf{y}_i - \bar{\mathbf{y}}(\tau))' V^{-1} (\mathbf{y}_i - \bar{\mathbf{y}}(\tau)), \qquad (11.19)$$

where V and $\bar{\mathbf{y}}(\tau)$ are estimated from the learning sample only.

After $R_\alpha(\mathcal{T})$ is defined, the rest of the procedure is identical to that in Section 4.2.3. We should mention, however, that a theoretical derivation of the standard error for $R(\mathcal{T})$ seems formidable. As a start, Zhang (1998a) suggested repeating the cross-validation procedure ten times. This process results in an empirical estimate of the needed standard error.

11.2.3 Computational Issues*

Because each node may have many possible splits, the homogeneity (11.15) must be computed a large number of times. Therefore, it is important to reduce the computational burden as much as possible by designing efficient algorithms. Computing $\mathbf{y}$ and w is relatively simple, so the critical part is to find $\hat{\Psi}$ and $\hat{\theta}$. To simplify the notation, we attach w to $\mathbf{y}$ and θ to Ψ and let

$$\mathbf{z} = (\mathbf{y}', w)' \text{ and } \Phi = (\Psi', \theta)'.$$

According to Fitzmaurice and Laird (1993), $\hat{\Phi}$ can be found through the following updating formulas:

$$\Phi^{(J+1)} = \Phi^{(J)} + V^{-1}(\mathbf{y})(\bar{\mathbf{y}} - I\!\!E\{\mathbf{Y}\}), \qquad (11.20)$$

where $I\!\!E\{\mathbf{Y}\}$ and $V^{-1}(\mathbf{y})$ are the mean and covariance matrix of $\mathbf{Y}$ given model parameters at $\Phi^{(J)}$, respectively, and $\bar{\mathbf{y}}$ is the sample average of $\mathbf{Y}$ within a given node. Not surprisingly, the computation of $V(\mathbf{Y})$ requires more time. Moreover, it depends on the current value $\Phi^{(J)}$ and makes the updating formula more vulnerable to a poor initial value of Φ. Both numerical and theoretical evidence suggests that it is better to replace the theoretical value of $V(\mathbf{Y})$ with the sample covariance matrix V_0 of $\mathbf{Y}$ within a given node. In our application, the use of V_0 leads to satisfactory numerical results. From a theoretical point of view, as $\Phi^{(J)}$ converges to a stable point and if the sample size is sufficiently large, $I\!\!E\{\mathbf{Y}\}$ and $V(\mathbf{Y})$ should be close to $\bar{\mathbf{y}}$ and V_0, respectively. So, the following simplified updating formula takes over the one in (11.20):

$$\Phi^{(J+1)} = \Phi^{(J)} + V_0^{-1}(\bar{\mathbf{y}} - I\!\!E\{\mathbf{Y}\}). \qquad (11.21)$$

11.2.4 Parameter Interpretation*

We have noted earlier that the canonical parameters correspond to conditional odds or odds ratios and that the conditions in these odds may not be appropriate. We illustrate here how to transform the canonical parameters to the marginal parameters that have natural interpretations.

Let $\gamma = I\!\!E(w)$ and $\boldsymbol{\mu} = (\mu_1, \ldots, \mu_q)' = I\!\!E(\mathbf{Y})$. Now we introduce an "overall" measure of pairwise correlations:

$$\rho = \frac{\gamma - \sum_{i<j} \mu_i \mu_j}{\sqrt{\sum_{i<j} \mu_i(1-\mu_i)\mu_j(1-\mu_j)}}. \qquad (11.22)$$

Next, we show how to derive the estimates of marginal distribution parameters, $\boldsymbol{\mu}$ and ρ, and their standard errors by making use of those of $\Phi = (\Psi', \theta)'$. The estimates for $\hat{\boldsymbol{\mu}}$ and $\hat{\rho}$ can be directly computed by substituting $\hat{\Phi}$ into the distribution function. What follows explains how to find the standard errors.

It is easy to see that

$$\frac{\partial \boldsymbol{\mu}}{\partial \Phi'} = \text{Cov}(\mathbf{Y}, \mathbf{Z}'), \text{ and } \frac{\partial \gamma}{\partial \Phi'} = \text{Cov}(w, \mathbf{Z}').$$

By the chain rule, we have

$$\begin{aligned}
\frac{\partial \rho}{\partial \Phi'} &= \frac{\partial \rho}{\partial \gamma} \frac{\partial \gamma}{\partial \Phi'} + \frac{\partial \rho}{\partial \boldsymbol{\mu}'} \frac{\partial \boldsymbol{\mu}}{\partial \Phi'} \\
&= \text{Cov}(w, \mathbf{Z}') \frac{\partial \rho}{\partial \gamma} + \frac{\partial \rho}{\partial \boldsymbol{\mu}'} \text{Cov}(\mathbf{Z}).
\end{aligned}$$

Therefore,

$$\begin{pmatrix} \frac{\partial \boldsymbol{\mu}}{\partial \boldsymbol{\Phi}'} \\ \frac{\partial \rho}{\partial \boldsymbol{\Phi}'} \end{pmatrix} = \begin{pmatrix} I & 0 \\ \frac{\partial \rho}{\partial \boldsymbol{\mu}'} & \frac{\partial \rho}{\partial \gamma} \end{pmatrix} \text{Cov}(\mathbf{z}) \stackrel{\text{def}}{=} JV.$$

Since V is the information matrix with respect to $\boldsymbol{\Phi}$, the information matrix for $\boldsymbol{\mu}$ and ρ is

$$\mathcal{I}(\boldsymbol{\mu}, \rho) = (VJ')^{-1} V (JV)^{-1} = (J^{-1})' V^{-1} J^{-1}.$$

Considering potential model misspecification as discussed by Fitzmaurice and Laird (1993) and Zhao and Prentice (1990), we should adopt a robust estimate for the covariance matrix of $\hat{\boldsymbol{\mu}}$ and $\hat{\rho}$ from Royall (1986) as follows:

$$\begin{aligned}
\hat{V}(\hat{\boldsymbol{\mu}}, \hat{\rho}) &= [n_\tau \mathcal{I}(\hat{\boldsymbol{\mu}}, \hat{\rho})]^{-1} \sum \left[(\hat{V}\hat{J}')^{-1} \begin{pmatrix} \mathbf{y}_i - \hat{\boldsymbol{\mu}} \\ w_i - \hat{\gamma} \end{pmatrix} \right. \\
&\qquad \left. \times \begin{pmatrix} \mathbf{y}_i - \hat{\boldsymbol{\mu}} \\ w_i - \hat{\gamma} \end{pmatrix}' (\hat{J}\hat{V})^{-1} \right] [n_\tau \mathcal{I}(\hat{\boldsymbol{\mu}}, \hat{\rho})]^{-1} \\
&= \frac{1}{n_\tau^2} \hat{J} \sum \begin{pmatrix} \mathbf{y}_i - \hat{\boldsymbol{\mu}} \\ w_i - \hat{\gamma} \end{pmatrix} \begin{pmatrix} \mathbf{y}_i - \hat{\boldsymbol{\mu}} \\ w_i - \hat{\gamma} \end{pmatrix}' \hat{J}',
\end{aligned}$$

where n_τ is the number of subjects in node τ and the summation is over all subjects in node τ. From the formula above it is numerically straightforward to compute the standard errors for $\hat{\boldsymbol{\mu}}$ and $\hat{\rho}$.

11.3 Application: Analysis of BROCS Data

11.3.1 Background

Building-related occupant complaint syndrome (BROCS) is a nonspecific set of related symptoms of discomfort reported by occupants of buildings. It occurs throughout the world in office buildings, hospitals, etc. The most common symptoms of BROCS include irritation of the eyes, nose, and throat; headache; and nausea. The cause of BROCS is generally not known. To enhance the understanding of BROCS, Zhang (1998a) analyzed a subset of the data from a 1989 survey of 6,800 employees of the Library of Congress and the headquarters of the Environmental Protection Agency in the United States. The discussion here is similar to the analysis of Zhang (1998a). In his analysis, Zhang built trees using the entire sample. But in order to validate the trees, we divide the sample equally into two sets: one to build the tree and one to validate it. Again, we also considered 22 predictors as the risk factors of BROCS (represented by 22 questions in Table 11.1) and 6 binary responses (each of which includes a number of specific health discomforts as given in Table 11.2). The purpose is to predict the risk of BROCS by identifying contributing factors.

TABLE 11.1. Explanatory Variables in the Study of BROCS

Predictor	Questions
x_1	What is the type of your working space? (enclosed office with door, cubicles, stacks, etc.)
x_2	How is your working space shared? (single, occupant, shared, etc.)
x_3	Do you have a metal desk? (yes or no)
x_4	Do you have new equipment at your work area? (yes or no)
x_5	Are you allergic to pollen? (yes or no)
x_6	Are you allergic to dust? (yes or no)
x_7	Are you allergic to molds? (yes or no)
x_8	How old are you? (16 to 70 years old)
x_9	Gender (male or female)
x_{10}	Is there too much air movement at your work area? (never, rarely, sometimes, often, always)
x_{11}	Is there too little air movement at your work area? (never, rarely, sometimes, often, always)
x_{12}	Is your work area too dry? (never, rarely, sometimes, often, always)
x_{13}	Is the air too stuffy at your work area? (never, rarely, sometimes, often, always)
x_{14}	Is your work area too noisy? (never, rarely, sometimes, often, always)
x_{15}	Is your work area too dusty? (never, rarely, sometimes, often, always)
x_{16}	Do you experience glare at your workstation? (no, sometimes, often, always)
x_{17}	How comfortable is your chair? (reasonably, somewhat, very uncomfortable, no one specific chair)
x_{18}	Is your chair easily adjustable? (yes, no, not adjustable)
x_{19}	Do you have influence over arranging the furniture? (very little, little, moderate, much, very much)
x_{20}	Do you have children at home? (yes or no)
x_{21}	Do you have major childcare duties? (yes or no)
x_{22}	What type of job do you have? (managerial, professional, technical, etc.)

This table is reproduced from Table 1 of Zhang (1998a).

TABLE 11.2. Six Clusters of BROCS

Response	Cluster	Included Symptoms
y_1	CNS	difficulty remembering/concentrating, dizziness, lightheadedness, depression, tension, nervousness
y_2	Upper Airway	runny/stuffy nose, sneezing, cough, sore throat
y_3	Pain	aching muscles/joints, pain in back/shoulders/neck, pain in hands/wrists
y_4	Flu-like	nausea, chills, fever
y_5	Eyes	dry, itching, or tearing eyes, sore/strained eyes, blurry vision, burning eyes
y_6	Lower Airway	wheezing in chest, shortness of breath, chest tightness

This table is reproduced from Table 2 of Zhang (1998a).

11.3.2 Tree Construction

Since some of the predictors have missing information, the missings together strategy described in Section 4.8.1 is adopted in the tree construction. To ensure that there is a reasonable number of subjects in every node, taking into account both the study sample size and the number of responses, Zhang (1998a) suggested not partitioning any node that has fewer than 60 subjects. In addition, the entire sample is equally divided into a learning and a validation sample in order to assess the performance of various approaches. The learning sample is used to construct trees and the validation sample to compare the predictive power of the constructed trees.

When $h(\tau)$ in (11.15) is used as a measure of node homogeneity, we obtained an initial tree with 65 nodes. Applying $R(\mathcal{T})$ defined in (11.18) as the tree cost, we derived a sequence of 33 nested optimal subtrees from the initial tree. Figure 11.2(a) plots the log cost of these subtrees against their complexity. In contrast, the use of $h_2(\tau)$ in (11.17) results in a starting tree of 199 nodes. Then, we obtained a sequence of 69 nested optimal subtrees using $R_2(\mathcal{T})$ in (11.19) as the tree cost. See Figure 11.2(b).

The subtree cost estimate and its standard error were derived from ten repetitions of 5-fold cross-validation. Each time, we have a 5-fold cross-validation estimate of the cost for every subtree. Repeating ten times gives ten such estimates. The average and the square root of the sample variance of these ten estimates are used as the tree cost estimate and its standard error, respectively. Based on Figure 11.2, we selected a 6-terminal-node final subtree from the initial tree using $h(\tau)$ shown in Figure 11.3 and a 7-terminal-node final subtree from the other initial tree depicted in Figure 11.4.

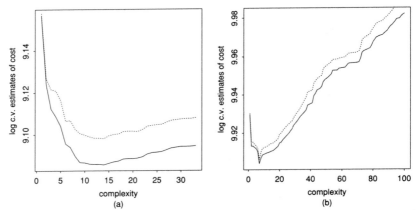

FIGURE 11.2. Cost-complexity for two sequences of nested subtrees. Panels (a) and (b) come from trees using $h(\tau)$ and $h_2(\tau)$, respectively. The solid line is the log cross-validation (CV) estimates of cost, and the dotted line is the log of one standard error above the estimated cost estimated by cross-validation.

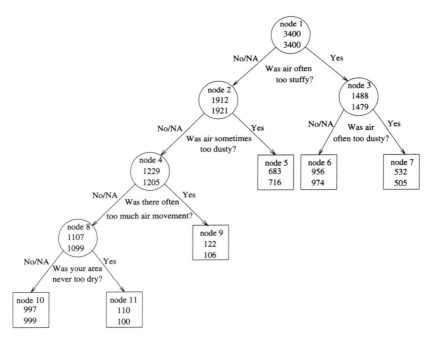

FIGURE 11.3. Tree structure for the risk factors of BROCS based on $h(\tau)$. Inside each node (a circle or a box) are the node number and the numbers of subjects in the learning (middle) and validation (bottom) samples. The splitting question is given under the node.

11.3 Application: Analysis of BROCS Data   191

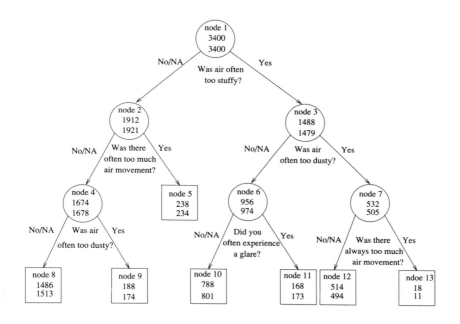

FIGURE 11.4. Tree structure for the risk factors of BROCS based on $h_2(\tau)$. Inside each node (a circle or a box) are the node number and the numbers of subjects in the learning (middle) and validation (bottom) samples. The splitting question is given under the node.

TABLE 11.3. Estimates of Symptom Prevalence Rates in the Terminal Nodes of the Tree in Figure 11.3

Terminal node #	Cluster of symptoms					
	CNS	U.A.	Pain	Flu-like	Eyes	L.A.
5	0.14[†]	0.29	0.29	0.15	0.03	0.10
	0.14[¶]	0.24	0.24	0.14	0.02	0.08
6	0.21	0.30	0.35	0.16	0.05	0.07
	0.20	0.31	0.35	0.19	0.05	0.07
7	0.29	0.49	0.51	0.29	0.08	0.12
	0.27	0.49	0.47	0.25	0.06	0.11
9	0.10	0.19	0.16	0.15	0.02	0.27
	0.08	0.20	0.17	0.13	0.01	0.18
10	0.07	0.09	0.10	0.06	0.01	0.03
	0.07	0.11	0.12	0.06	0.01	0.02
11	0.21	0.26	0.24	0.17	0.05	0.09
	0.08	0.14	0.26	0.08	0.04	0.04

[†]Based on the learning sample.
[¶]Based on the validation sample.

11.3.3 Description of Numerical Results

Table 11.3 suggests that terminal node 7 in Figure 11.3 is most troublesome. Subjects in this terminal node complained about more problems in nearly all clusters than everyone else. This is because the air quality in their working area was poor, namely, often too stuffy and dusty. For the same reasons, subjects in terminal nodes 5 and 6 also reported relatively more symptoms. In contrast, subjects in terminal node 10 experienced the least discomfort because they had the best air quality. Overall, Figure 11.3 and Table 11.3 show the importance of air quality around the working area.

Based on a different criterion, $h_2(\tau)$, Figure 11.4 demonstrates again the importance of air quality. It uses nearly the same splits as Figure 11.3 except that "experiencing a glare" also emerged as a splitting factor. By comparing terminal nodes 10 and 11 in Figure 11.4, it appears that "experiencing a glare" resulted in more discomfort for all clusters of symptoms.

11.3.4 Alternative Approaches

We mention two alternative approaches that make direct use of the tree methods for a single outcome as described in earlier chapters. First, we could grow separate trees for individual clusters of symptoms and then attempt to summarize the information. Depending on the number of clusters, this approach could be very laborious and not necessarily as productive, as explained by Zhang (1998a). The second approach is to create a surrogate response variable. This surrogate response can be taken as the sum of the

TABLE 11.4. Estimates of Symptom Prevalence Rates in the Terminal Nodes of the Tree in Figure 11.4

Terminal node #	Cluster of symptoms					
	CNS	U.A.	Pain	Flu-like	Eyes	L.A.
5	0.15†	0.27	0.27	0.21	0.04	0.24
	0.12¶	0.25	0.26	0.18	0.02	0.21
8	0.09	0.13	0.14	0.08	0.01	0.04
	0.08	0.14	0.15	0.07	0.01	0.03
9	0.16	0.41	0.34	0.20	0.04	0.10
	0.18	0.29	0.28	0.17	0.01	0.05
10	0.19	0.29	0.30	0.13	0.04	0.06
	0.18	0.30	0.32	0.16	0.04	0.06
11	0.31	0.36	0.57	0.28	0.10	0.08
	0.28	0.37	0.51	0.30	0.08	0.08
12	0.28	0.48	0.51	0.28	0.08	0.10
	0.27	0.49	0.47	0.25	0.06	0.11
13	0.56	0.61	0.44	0.56	0.22	0.61
	0.18	0.45	0.36	0.18	0.18	0.27

†Based on the learning sample.
¶Based on the validation sample.

positive responses in the six clusters or a more sophisticated linear combination derived from a descriptive principal components analysis (Kleinbaum, 1988, p. 604). It is regarded as descriptive because the responses are binary, which do not satisfy the conditions of principal components analysis. Then, we can treat the surrogate response as a numerical variable and grow a regression tree for it. After such a regression tree is grown, we can regard it as a classification tree for the original binary outcomes. We refer to Zhang (1998a) for details.

11.3.5 Predictive Performance

To compare the predictive performance of the trees constructed in Figures 11.3 and 11.4, we produce ROC curves (see Section 3.2 for the description of ROC curves) for individual clusters. Figure 11.5 displays two sets of ROC curves: one from the prediction rule based on Figure 11.3 and the other on Figure 11.4. In addition, the areas under the ROC curves are listed. Each panel of Figure 11.5 corresponds to a cluster. The performance of the two trees is very close, as indicated by both the ROC curves and the areas under the curves, although Figure 11.4 is decisively better than Figure 11.3 for the clusters of "flu-like" and "lower airway."

194   11. Analysis of Multiple Discrete Responses

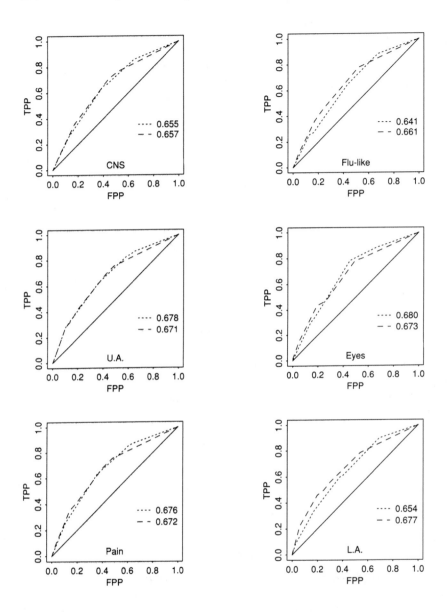

FIGURE 11.5. Comparison of ROC curves for the classifications tree in Figures 11.3 and 11.4 among individual clusters. The true positive probability (TPP) is plotted against the false positive probability (FPP). The solid line indicates the performance of a random prediction. The dotted and dashed ROC curves respectively come from Figures 11.3 and 11.4, and the areas under them are also reported.

11.4 Polytomous and Longitudinal Responses

The homogeneity $h(\tau)$ can be further extended to analyze longitudinal binary responses and polytomous responses. For longitudinal data, the time trend can be incorporated into the parameters introduced in (11.14), hence allowing $h(\tau)$ to be a function of time. For polytomous responses, additional parameters corresponding to various levels of the outcomes can be included in (11.14). For instance, the component $\Psi'\mathbf{y}$ in (11.14) can be replaced with

$$\sum_{k=1}^{q}\sum_{l=1}^{c_k-1}\psi_{kl}I(y_k>l)$$

or

$$\sum_{k=1}^{q}\sum_{l=1}^{c_k-1}\psi_{kl}I(y_k=l),$$

depending on whether or not the outcomes are ordinal, where c_k is the number of levels for y_k, $k=1,\ldots,q$, and $I(\cdot)$ is the indicator function. It is also easy to see that all outcomes do not have to have the same number of categories nor must they be of the same type (some ordinal and some nominal outcomes are allowed). Nevertheless, the implementation of these ideas requires substantial computational effort.

11.5 Analysis of the BROCS Data via Log-Linear Models

Building a log-linear model with standard software such as SAS and SPLUS is usually a prohibitive task when we include a large number of factors into the model and consider their higher-order interactions. In the present application, given the six response variables it is not realistic to scrutinize all 22 covariates in the same model. In fact, it was still computationally too ambitious when we entered only four variables (in their original scale) that appeared in Figures 11.3 and 11.4. As a compromise, we dichotomized the four variables based on the splits and created four dummy variables: $z_1=I(x_{10}>3)$, $z_2=I(x_{12}>3)$, $z_3=I(x_{13}>3)$, and $z_4=I(x_{15}>3)$. In log-linear models, we assume that the sample counts for the 2^{10} cross-classification cells of y's and z's are independent Poisson random variables with expected values to be modeled.

We started with a model that allows for third-order interactions between two of the 6 response variables and one of the 4 dummy variables. The first `PROC CATMOD` statement of the SAS program in Table 11.5 carried out the estimation for the initial model. Insignificant terms (p-value ≥ 0.05) were removed from the model sequentially, which led to the final log-linear model with the expected cell counts specified by

$$\exp\left[\mu + \sum_{k=1}^{6} \lambda_{i_k}^{y_k} + \sum_{k=1}^{4} \lambda_{j_k}^{z_k}\right.$$
$$+ \left(\sum_{k=4,6} \lambda_{j_1 i_k}^{z_1 y_k} + \sum_{k \neq 3,5} \lambda_{j_2 i_k}^{z_2 y_k} + \sum_{k \neq 2,5} \lambda_{j_3 i_k}^{z_3 y_k} + \sum_{k=1}^{4} \lambda_{j_4 i_k}^{z_4 y_k}\right)$$
$$+ \left(\sum_{l=1,2} \sum_{k=3}^{6} \lambda_{i_l i_k}^{y_l y_k} + \sum_{k=4}^{6} \lambda_{i_3 i_k}^{y_3 y_k} + \sum_{k=5}^{6} \lambda_{i_4 i_k}^{y_4 y_k} + \lambda_{i_5 i_6}^{y_5 y_6}\right)$$
$$\left. + \left(\lambda_{j_2 i_2 i_4}^{z_2 y_2 y_4} + \sum_{k=4,6} \lambda_{j_3 i_3 i_k}^{z_3 y_3 y_k} + \sum_{k=1,3} \lambda_{j_4 i_k i_4}^{z_4 y_k y_4}\right)\right]. \quad (11.23)$$

The second PROC CATMOD statement of the SAS program in Table 11.5 performed the computation for model (11.23). The results were organized in Table 11.6 in five categories based on the grouping of the terms in model (11.23).

Interpreting Table 11.6 rigorously and thoroughly would be difficult and may be even impossible because of the mutual relationship among the responses and covariates. Our attempt here is merely to extract the major message in a descriptive manner. Table 11.6 confirms the correlation between the 6 response variables. Conditional on everything else, the first response variable (CNS) appears to be uncorrelated with the second (upper airway) response because the final model does not contain the interaction: $y_1 * y_2$. Five of the 14 significant correlations between the 6 responses may be mediated by the three dummy variables z_2 to z_4. The dummy variable z_1 (air movement) has significant effects only on the mean frequency of the fourth (flu-like) and sixth (lower airway) clusters of symptoms. The air dryness (z_2) may not be significantly associated with the pain (y_3) and lower airway (y_6) symptoms. Although we have seen the importance of air stuffiness (z_3) in the tree-based analysis, the log-linear model does not suggest that it significantly affects the upper airway (y_2) and eye (y_5) problems. Finally, the dusty air (z_4) did not express significant association with the eye (y_5) and lower airway (y_6) symptoms although we expect that the dusty air would cause more eye discomfort. One might think that relatively few reports in the eye cluster perhaps limited our power; however, the model reveals its significant association with air dryness. One good explanation comes from the tree in Figure 11.4, where we see that the combination of dusty air with movement resulted in many more eye problems. Due to practical limitations, it was not possible to consider the interactions between the covariates in the initial model. As a matter of fact, the interaction,

11.5 Analysis of the BROCS Data via Log-Linear Models

TABLE 11.5. SAS Program for the Analysis of BROCS Data

```
data one;
infile 'BROCS.DAT';
input x1-x22 y1-y6;
run;
data two; set one;
where x10 ne . and x12 ne . and x13 ne . and x15 ne .;
z1 = (x10 > 3); z2 = (x12 > 3);
z3 = (x13 > 3); z4 = (x15 > 3);
proc sort; by z1 z2 z3 z4 y1 y2 y3 y4 y6;
proc freq noprint;
    tables z1*z2*z3*z4*y1*y2*y3*y4*y5*y6
           /list out=counts;
run;
proc catmod data=counts; weight count;
model z1*z2*z3*z4*y1*y2*y3*y4*y5*y6 = _response_
    /ml noprofile noresponse noiter;
loglin y1|y2|z1 y1|y2|z2 y1|y2|z3 y1|y2|z4
       y1|y3|z1 y1|y3|z2 y1|y3|z3 y1|y3|z4
       y1|y4|z1 y1|y4|z2 y1|y4|z3 y1|y4|z4
       y1|y5|z1 y1|y5|z2 y1|y5|z3 y1|y5|z4
       y1|y6|z1 y1|y6|z2 y1|y6|z3 y1|y6|z4
       y2|y3|z1 y2|y3|z2 y2|y3|z3 y2|y3|z4
       y2|y4|z1 y2|y4|z2 y2|y4|z3 y2|y4|z4
       y2|y5|z1 y2|y5|z2 y2|y5|z3 y2|y5|z4
       y2|y6|z1 y2|y6|z2 y2|y6|z3 y2|y6|z4
       y3|y4|z1 y3|y4|z2 y3|y4|z3 y3|y4|z4
       y3|y5|z1 y3|y5|z2 y3|y5|z3 y3|y5|z4
       y3|y6|z1 y3|y6|z2 y3|y6|z3 y3|y6|z4
       y4|y5|z1 y4|y5|z2 y4|y5|z3 y4|y5|z4
       y4|y6|z1 y4|y6|z2 y4|y6|z3 y4|y6|z4
       y5|y6|z1 y5|y6|z2 y5|y6|z3 y5|y6|z4;
run;
proc catmod data=counts; weight count;
model z1*z2*z3*z4*y1*y2*y3*y4*y5*y6 = _response_
    /ml noprofile noresponse noiter;

loglin y1*z2 y1*z3 y2*z4 y1*y3 y2*y3 y4*z1 y5*z2
       y2*y5 y3*y5 y1|y4|z4 y1|y5 y1|y6 y6|z1
       y2|y4|z2 y2|y6 y3|y4|z3 y3|y4|z4 y3|y6|z3
       y4|y5 y4|y6 y5|y6;
run;
```

TABLE 11.6. SAS Program for the Analysis of BROCS Data

Effect	Estimate	Error	Prob.	Effect	Estimate	Error	Prob.
Y1	0.218	0.049	0.0000	Y2	−0.212	0.055	0.0001
Y3	−0.230	0.058	0.0001	Y4	0.137	0.055	0.0125
Y5	1.116	0.054	0.0000	Y6	0.427	0.053	0.0000
Z1	0.604	0.030	0.0000	Z2	0.019	0.038	0.6161
Z3	−0.103	0.029	0.0004	Z4	0.322	0.022	0.0000
Z1*Y4	0.112	0.028	0.0001	Z1*Y6	0.421	0.028	0.0000
Z2*Y1	0.117	0.019	0.0000	Z2*Y2	0.157	0.019	0.0000
Z2*Y4	0.080	0.020	0.0000	Z2*Y5	0.137	0.038	0.0002
Z3*Y1	0.146	0.020	0.0000	Z3*Y3	0.106	0.028	0.0001
Z3*Y4	0.100	0.021	0.0000	Z3*Y6	−0.090	0.026	0.0007
Z4*Y1	0.068	0.022	0.0016	Z4*Y2	0.214	0.018	0.0000
Z4*Y3	0.085	0.022	0.0001	Z4*Y4	0.090	0.022	0.0001
Y1*Y3	0.210	0.020	0.0000	Y1*Y4	0.277	0.023	0.0000
Y1*Y5	0.202	0.043	0.0000	Y1*Y6	0.166	0.031	0.0000
Y2*Y3	0.345	0.017	0.0000	Y2*Y4	0.137	0.022	0.0000
Y2*Y5	0.290	0.047	0.0000	Y2*Y6	0.157	0.030	0.0000
Y3*Y4	0.189	0.023	0.0000	Y3*Y5	0.197	0.050	0.0001
Y3*Y6	0.088	0.032	0.0053	Y4*Y5	0.127	0.047	0.0061
Y4*Y6	0.250	0.032	0.0000	Y5*Y6	0.257	0.052	0.0000
Z2*Y2*Y4	0.079	0.019	0.0000				
Z3*Y3*Y4	0.063	0.020	0.0015	Z3*Y3*Y6	0.111	0.026	0.0000
Z4*Y1*Y4	0.067	0.021	0.0018	Z4*Y3*Y4	0.093	0.020	0.0000

11.5 Analysis of the BROCS Data via Log-Linear Models

$z_2 * z_4 * y_5$, would be extremely significant if we knew that it should be included.

In retrospect, log-linear models provide us with the opportunity to explore the association among many categorical variables. Due to the model's complexity, we are usually confined to simplistic choices of log-linear models and have to give up the chance of exploring some important relationships. The tree-based analysis offers a fruitful complement to the use of log-linear models, particularly in dimension reduction and model specification.

12
Appendix

In this chapter we provide some script files that show how to run the RTREE program and how to read the output resulting from the execution of the program. The analysis presented in Chapter 2 results from these files.

12.1 The Script for Running RTREE Automatically

To run the RTREE program, simply execute the program after downloading it and then enter your inputs following the online instructions. A few simple inputs are required from the user. We shaded the user inputs in the script files to distinguish them from the other texts.

The illustration here assumes that a data set, named `example.dat`, is saved in the same directory as the RTREE program. The user is asked to enter the data file name. As introduced in Chapter 4, there are various node-splitting criteria. The RTREE adopts either the entropy impurity or the Gini index. The program can be run automatically or manually. The user needs to specify the execution mode. If automatic mode is chosen, no further question will be asked and the program creates two files, `example.inf` and `example.ps`, in the same directory. We will explain the `example.inf` file shortly, and Figure 2.3 is made from the `example.ps` file.

12. Appendix

```
----------This is the script file of running RTREE automatically----------
==================================================================
*This RTREE program implements the ideas expressed in:           *
*1. Zhang and Bracken (1995) Amer. J. of Epidemio., 141, 70-78.  *
*2. Zhang, Holford, and Bracken (1995) Statistics in Medicine,   *
*   15, 37-50.                                                   *
*This program is meant to be a research tool, and the users are  *
*responsible for the correctness of their own analysis. Also,    *
*please send emails to:                                          *
*              heping.zhang@yale.edu                             *
*should you find any bugs or have any suggestions. If you use    *
*this program for your work, it is understood (a) that you will  *
*keep the author of this program informed and (b) that you will  *
*refer to this program as RTREE, not any other names.Thank you.  *
*@Copyrighted by Heping Zhang, 1997. Distribution not limited.   *
*Last updated on April 28, 1998.                                 *
==================================================================

Please input datafile name: example.dat
Choose splitting rule [enter 1 for entropy(default) or 2 for
gini]: 1
       For new users, it is important to read the following ...
==================================================================
*The tree is initialized. You will be asked whether you want to *
*control the tree construction process. For the first time, I   *
*would recommend you not controlling it. Instead, let the       *
*program run automatically. In that case, you should enter      *
*n as your answer. Both initial and pruned trees will be saved  *
*in a file:               example.inf.                          *
*If you wish, you can print the tree output and use it as a     *
*reference to rerun the program at the controlled mode by       *
*entering y as your answer.                                     *
==================================================================
*WARNING: If you don't want the file b3.inf to be overwritten,
use Ctrl-C to exit immediately.

!!!!!!!!!!!!!!!!!!!!!!   Now, enjoy  !!!!!!!!!!!!!!!!!!!!!!!!!

Do you want to control the splitting [y/n(default)]? n

An initial tree with 129 nodes is grown, ready to prune
Prune is finished. There remain 13 nodes.
Ready to draw PS file.
Please view or print PS file: b3.ps
Press Enter to end this program!
```

12.2 The Script for Running RTREE Manually

Understandably, running the RTREE program manually requires better knowledge of the method than doing it automatically. On the other hand, it provides us with an important opportunity to incorporate our scientific judgment into the data analysis without compromising statistical principle. Because of the stepwise nature of the tree-based method, the manual mode allows the user to explore alternative tree structures, leading to trees of better quality; See, e.g., Zhang (1998b). We recommend reading Chapter 4 before running the program in the manual mode.

During the course of execution, the user is asked whether a node needs to be split. If the answer is yes, a computer-selected split is presented for the user's consideration. The split can be accepted, or the computer pops up a list of the best candidate splits from all predictor variables. Although Table 2.1 contains 15 variables, the script file here lists 22 variables. This is because there are 7 ordinal or continuous variables that have missing values. Thus, seven new variables are created, as discussed in Section 4.8.1. Those best candidate splits are ordered according to their numerical quality, and any of them can be chosen by entering the corresponding rank. Then some information with regard to the properties of the chosen split is printed on the screen. If none of the suggested splits is desirable, a completely new split can be enforced. But the user should be familiar with the variable names and distributions and be ready to enter the split. Read and follow the online instructions for the input. If the user is ready to stop splitting, simply answer no to all questions that ask whether a node should be split.

12. Appendix

```
----------This is the script file of running RTREE automatically----------
==================================================================
*This RTREE program implements the ideas expressed in:           *
*1. Zhang and Bracken (1995) Amer. J. of Epidemio., 141, 70-78.*
*2. Zhang, Holford, and Bracken (1995) Statistics in Medicine, *
*   15, 37-50.                                                    *
*This program is meant to be a research tool, and the users are*
*responsible for the correctness of their own analysis. Also,   *
*please send emails to:                                          *
*                heping.zhang@yale.edu                           *
*should you find any bugs or have any suggestions. If you use   *
*this program for your work, it is understood (a) that you will*
*keep the author of this program informed and (b) that you will*
*refer to this program as RTREE, not any other names.Thank you.*
*@Copyrighted by Heping Zhang, 1997. Distribution not limited.  *
*Last updated on April 28, 1998.                                 *
==================================================================


Please input datafile name: example.dat
Choose splitting rule [enter 1 for entropy(default) or 2 for
gini]: 1
      For new users, it is important to read the following ...
==================================================================
*The tree is initialized. You will be asked whether you want to*
*control the tree construction process. For the first time, I  *
*would recommend you not controlling it. Instead, let the       *
*program run automatically. In that case, you should enter     *
*n as your answer. Both initial and pruned trees will be saved *
*in a file:              example.inf.                           *
*If you wish, you can print the tree output and use it as a    *
*reference to rerun the program at the controlled mode by      *
*entering y as your answer.                                     *
==================================================================
*WARNING: If you don't want the file b3.inf to be overwritten,
use Ctrl-C to exit immediately.

!!!!!!!!!!!!!!!!!!!!   Now, enjoy   !!!!!!!!!!!!!!!!!!!!!!!!!!

Do you want to control the splitting [y/n(default)]? y

3861 cases in node 1.  Split [y/n]? y
The impurity of the split=0.203560
The resubstitution relative risk=2.301200 and
   its 95 percent confidence interval=(1.703034, 3.109462)
A 5-fold cross validation relative risk=2.143026 and
   its 95 percent confidence interval=(1.586902, 2.894042)
This split uses categorical variable 3 and a case
goes to right for category[ies]
2
Accept this split [y/n]? y
3151 cases in node 2.  Split [y/n]? y
The impurity of the split=0.175190
The resubstitution relative risk=2.510655 and
   its 95 percent confidence interval=(1.472348, 4.281182)
A 5-fold cross validation relative risk=2.525424 and
   its 95 percent confidence interval=(1.480783, 4.307023)
This split uses ordinal variable 11 and a case goes to right
if greater than 4.000000
```

```
Accept this split [y/n]? y
710 cases in node 3.  Split [y/n]? y
The impurity of the split=0.317509
The resubstitution relative risk=2.074219 and
   its 95 percent confidence interval=(1.065797, 4.036776)
A 5-fold cross validation relative risk=1.131193 and
   its 95 percent confidence interval=(0.676505, 1.891481)
This split uses categorical variable 7 and a case
goes to right for category[ies]
1
Accept this split [y/n]? y
2980 cases in node 4.  Split [y/n]? y
The impurity of the split=0.165181
The resubstitution relative risk=3.480179 and
   its 95 percent confidence interval=(1.615488, 7.497205)
A 5-fold cross validation relative risk=1.274209 and
   its 95 percent confidence interval=(0.833830, 1.947168)
This split uses categorical variable 12 and a case
goes to right for category[ies]
4,1,0
Accept this split [y/n]? n
rank: impurity variable no.
    1: 0.16518   12
    2: 0.16568   17
    3: 0.16569   6
    4: 0.16580   1
    5: 0.16610   14
    6: 0.16618   15
    7: 0.16618   22
    8: 0.16632   9
    9: 0.16632   18
   10: 0.16633   2
   11: 0.16637   21
   12: 0.16638   16
   13: 0.16640   5
   14: 0.16643   11
   15: 0.16643   19
   16: 0.16653   10
   17: 0.16657   8
   18: 0.16657   4
   19: 0.16659   13
   20: 0.16659   20
   21: 0.16660   7
   22: 0.16665   3
which one [enter the rank number, 0 for none of the above]?
0
Do you still want to split this node [y/n]? 0
which variable [enter the variable number]: 0
This variable has 6 categories:
0 1 2 3 4 -9
Enter a sequence of 6 0's and 1's to specify the split.
For example, 1 1 0 0 0 0 sends the first two categories to one
side and the rest to the other side.
Enter here: 0 0 1 1 0 0
The impurity of the split=0.164899
The resubstitution relative risk=5.096198 and
   its 95 percent confidence interval=(2.049671, 12.670928)
A 5-fold cross validation relative risk=1.823560 and
```

```
    its 95 percent confidence interval=(0.932500, 3.566081)
171 cases in node 5.   Split [y/n]? n
no split for node 5:2
512 cases in node 6.   Split [y/n]? n
no split for node 6:2
198 cases in node 7.   Split [y/n]? n
no split for node 7:2
31 cases in node 8.    Split [y/n]? n
no split for node 8:2
2949 cases in node 9.  Split [y/n]? n
no split for node 9:2
There remain 9 nodes.
Ready to draw PS file.
Please view or print PS file: example.ps
Press Enter to end this program!
```

12.3 The .inf File

This is the .inf output file from the RTREE program running in automatic mode. It has three parts. The first part checks and summarizes the variables. The second part provides information regarding the large tree before pruning, and the last part is for the pruned tree. The formats for the last two parts are the same. Their six columns are (i) node number (node 1 is the root node); (ii) number of subjects in the node; (iii) left daughter node number; (iv) right daughter node number; (v) the node-splitting variable; and (vi) the splitting value corresponds to the node-splitting variable for an internal node or the numbers of 0 and 1 outcomes in a terminal node. For an internal node, a floating value is for a continuous or ordinal variable and a set of integers for a nominal variable. Figure 2.3 is a graphical presentation of the information from the last part of this file.

12. Appendix

------------------------------This is the .inf file----------------------------
```
There are 15 covariates
Original status of variables are
1 3 3 3 1 1 3 3 1 3 1 3 1 1 1
1 refers to an ordinal covariate and a positive integer
i means a nominal one that has i categories.
For an ordinal covariate, the min. and max. will be given;
For a nominal one, the counts corresponding to each level
will be listed.
 1: 13.000000 46.000000
 2: 3017(1) 68(2) 69(3) 1(4) 703(5) 3(-9)
 3: 3008(1) 710(2) 109(3) 21(4) 6(5) 7(-9)
 4: 3488(0) 369(1) 4(-9)
 5: 1.000000 9.000000
 6: 4.000000 27.000000
 7: 1521(0) 1957(1) 1(2) 382(-9)
 8: 1116(0) 1221(1) 1524(-9)
 9: 0.000000 66.000000
10: 2146(0) 1700(1) 15(-9)
11: 1.000000 10.000000
12: 3072(0) 30(1) 32(2) 1(3) 680(4) 46(-9)
13: 0.000000 3.000000
14: 12.600000 1273.000000
15: 0.000000 7.000000

The initial tree:
  node  #cases   left   right  split var     cutoff
    1    3861      2       3       3          {2}
    2    3151      4       5      11         4.00000
    3     710      6       7       7          {1}
    4    2980      8       9      12        {4,1,0}
    5     171     10      11       6        15.00000
    6     512     12      13       1        26.00000
    7     198     14      15      10          {0}
    8      61 terminal node with distribution: 53 8
    9    2919     16      17       6        12.00000/NA
   10     127     18      19       7          {1}
   11      44 terminal node with distribution: 43 1
   12     443     20      21      14        45.50000
   13      69 terminal node with distribution: 65 4
   14     120     22      23      14       187.20000/NA
   15      78     24      25      14        12.60000
   16     983     26      27      14        12.60000/NA
   17    1936     28      29       1        32.00000
   18      83     30      31      14       187.20000/NA
   19      44 terminal node with distribution: 35 9
   20     258     32      33       1        19.00000
   21     185     34      35       7          {0}
   22      61 terminal node with distribution: 58 3
   23      59 terminal node with distribution: 59 0
   24      39 terminal node with distribution: 32 7
   25      39 terminal node with distribution: 38 1
   26      43 terminal node with distribution: 43 0
   27     940     36      37      15         1.00000
   28    1602     38      39       1        30.00000
   29     334     40      41      14       174.60001/NA
   30      43 terminal node with distribution: 37 6
   31      40 terminal node with distribution: 39 1
   32     130     42      43       1        17.00000
```

---------------------------The .inf file continued---------------------------
```
33      128      44         45      13      0.00000
34       47 terminal node with distribution: 35 12
35      138      46         47      15      0.00000
36      772      48         49       6     11.00000
36      772      48         49       6     11.00000
37      168      50         51      14    307.50000/NA
38     1320      52         53      15      1.00000
39      282      54         55      15      0.00000
40      206      56         57       6     16.00000
41      128      58         59      15      0.00000
42       61 terminal node with distribution: 57 4
43       69 terminal node with distribution: 56 13
44       59 terminal node with distribution: 57 2
45       69 terminal node with distribution: 61 8
46       46 terminal node with distribution: 37 9
47       92      60         61      14    133.50000
48      177      62         63       7       {0}
49      595      64         65      10       {1}
50      119      66         67      14    101.60000
51       49 terminal node with distribution: 48 1
52     1223      68         69      14    147.00000/NA
53       97      70         71       8      {1,0}
54       95      72         73      14    147.00000/NA
55      187 terminal node with distribution: 187 0
56      102      74         75       6     15.00000
57      104      76         77      14     75.60000
58       50 terminal node with distribution: 48 2
59       78 terminal node with distribution: 78 0
60       45 terminal node with distribution: 39 6
61       47 terminal node with distribution: 46 1
62       75 terminal node with distribution: 65 10
63      102      78         79       6     10.00000
64      235      80         81      14     14.10000
65      360      82         83      14    378.00000/NA
66       62 terminal node with distribution: 58 4
67       57 terminal node with distribution: 48 9
68      660      84         85       9     14.00000
69      563      86         87       6     15.00000
70       44 terminal node with distribution: 38 6
71       53 terminal node with distribution: 53 0
```
(This second part is truncated from here to the end.)

The pruned tree:
```
  node  #cases    left    right  split var   cutoff
     1    3861       2       3        3        {2}
     2    3151       4       5       11       4.00000
     3     710       6       7        7        {1}
     4    2980       8       9       12      {4,1,0}
     5     171 terminal node with distribution: 154 17
     6     512 terminal node with distribution: 453 59
     7     198 terminal node with distribution: 187 11
     8      61 terminal node with distribution: 53 8
     9    2919      16      17        6      12.00000/NA
    16     983 terminal node with distribution: 932 51
    17    1936      28      29        1      32.00000
    28    1602 terminal node with distribution: 1561 41
    29     334 terminal node with distribution: 316 18
```

References

[1] A. Agresti. *Categorical Data Analysis*. John Wiley & Sons, New York, 1990.

[2] N.S. Altman. An iterated Cochrane–Orcutt procedure for nonparametric regression. *Journal of Statistical Computation and Simulation*, 40:93–108, 1992.

[3] S.M. Ansell, B.L. Rapoport, G. Falkson, J.I. Raats, and C.M. Moeken. Survival determinants in patients with advanced ovarian cancer. *Gynecologic Oncology*, 50:215–220, 1993.

[4] A. Babiker and J. Cuzick. A simple frailty model for family studies with covariates. *Statistics in Medicine*, 13:1679–1692, 1994.

[5] P. Bacchetti and M.R. Segal. Survival trees with time-dependent covariates: application to estimating changes in the incubation period of aids. *Lifetime Data Analysis*, 1:35–47, 1995.

[6] R.R. Bahadur. A representation of the joint distribution of responses to n dichotomous items. In *Studies on Item Analysis and Prediction*, pages 158–168, Stanford, California, 1961. Stanford University Press.

[7] G.E. Bonney. Regression logistic models for familial disease and other binary traits. *Biometrics*, 42:611–625, 1986.

[8] G.E. Bonney. Logistic regression for dependent binary observations. *Biometrics*, 43:951–973, 1987.

References

[9] G.E. Box, G.M. Jenkins, and G.C. Reinsel. *Time Series Analysis*. Wiley, New York, 3rd edition, 1994.

[10] M.B. Bracken. *Perinatal Epidemiology*. Oxford University Press, New York, 1984.

[11] M.B. Bracken, K.G. Hellenbrand, T.R. Holford, and C. Bryce-Buchanan. Low birth weight in pregnancies following induced abortion: No evidence for an association. *American Journal of Epidemiology*, 123:604–613, 1986.

[12] M.B. Bracken, K. Belanger, K.G. Hellenbrand, et al. Exposure to electromagnetic fields during pregnancy with emphasis on electrically heated beds: association with birthweight and intrauterine growth retardation. *Epidemiology*, 6:263–270, 1995.

[13] L. Breiman, J.H. Friedman, R.A. Olshen, and C.J. Stone. *Classification and Regression Trees*. Wadsworth, California, 1984.

[14] N. Breslow. Contribution to the discussion of paper by D.R. Cox. *Journal of the Royal Statistical Society-B*, 34:216–217, 1972.

[15] R. Brookmeyer. Reconstruction and future trends of the AIDS epidemic in the united states. *Science*, 253:37–42, 1991.

[16] J. Buckley and I. James. Linear regression with censored data. *Biometrika*, 66:429–436, 1979.

[17] C. Cannings, E.A. Thompson, and M.H. Skolnick. Probability functions on complex pedigrees. *Advances in Applied Probability*, 10:26–61, 1978.

[18] D. Carmelli, J. Halpern, G.E. Swan, et al. 27-year mortality in the western collaborative group study: construction of risk groups by recursive partitioning. *Journal of Clinical Epidemiology*, 44:1341–1351, 1991.

[19] D. Carmelli, H.P. Zhang, and G.E. Swan. Obesity and 33 years of coronary heart disease and cancer mortality in the western collaborative group study. *Epidemiology*, 8:378–383, 1997.

[20] H. Chipman, E.I. George, and R. McCulloch. Bayesian CART model search. *Journal of the American Statistical Association*, 93:935–948, 1998.

[21] S.C. Choi, J.P. Muizelaar, T.Y. Barnes, et al. Prediction tree for severely head-injured patients. *Journal of Neurosurgery*, 75:251–255, 1991.

[22] P.A. Chou, T. Lookabaugh, and R.M. Gray. Optimal pruning with applications to tree-structured source coding and modeling. *IEEE Trans. Information Theory*, 35:299–315, 1989.

[23] A. Ciampi, A. Hogg, S. McKinney, and J. Thiffault. A computer program for recursive partition and amalgamation for censored survival data. *Computer Methods and Programs in Biomedicine*, 26:239–256, 1988.

[24] A. Ciampi, J. Thiffault, J.P. Nakache, and B. Asselain. Stratification by stepwise regression, correspondence analysis and recursive partition: A comparison of three methods of analysis for survival data with covariates. *Computational Statistics and Data Analysis*, 4:185–204, 1986.

[25] W.G. Cochran. Some methods of strengthening the common χ^2 test. *Biometrics*, 10:417–451, 1954.

[26] M.A. Connolly and K.Y. Liang. Conditional logistic regression models for correlated binary data. *Biometrika*, 75:501–506, 1988.

[27] P.C. Cosman, R.M. Gray, and R.A. Olshen. Vector quantization: Clustering and classification trees. *Proceedings of the IEEE*, 82:919–932, 1994.

[28] D.R. Cox. Regression models and life-tables (with discussion). *Journal of the Royal Statistical Society-B*, 34:187–220, 1972.

[29] D.R. Cox and E.J. Snell. *The Analysis of Binary Data*. Chapman and Hall, London, 2nd edition, 1989.

[30] P. Craven and G. Wahba. Smoothing noisy data with spline functions. *Numerical Mathematics*, 31:377–403, 1979.

[31] N. Cressie and S.N. Lahiri. The asymptotic distribution of REML estimators. *Journal of Multivariate Analysis*, 45:217–233, 1993.

[32] M.J. Crowder and D.J. Hand. *Analysis of Repeated Measures*. Chapman and Hall, London, 1990.

[33] J. Crowley, M. LeBlanc, R. Gentleman, and S. Salmon. Exploratory methods in survival analysis. In *IMS Lecture Notes—Monograph Series 27*, pages 55–77, H.L. Koul and J.V. Deshpande, eds. IMS, Hayward, CA, 1995.

[34] W.J. Curran, C.B. Scott, J. Horton, et al. Recursive partitioning analysis of prognostic factors in three radiation therapy oncology group malignant glioma trials. *Journal of the National Cancer Institute*, 85:704–710, 1993.

[35] J.R. Dale. Global cross-ratio models for bivariate, discrete, ordered responses. *Biometrics*, 42:909–917, 1986.

[36] R. Davis and J. Anderson. Exponential survival trees. *Statistics in Medicine*, 8:947–962, 1989.

[37] T.R. Dawber. *The Framingham Study: The Epidemiology of Atherosclerotic Disease*. Harvard University Press, Cambridge, 1980.

[38] A.P. Dempster, N.M. Laird, and D.B. Rubin. Maximum likelihood from incomplete data via the EM algorithm. *Journal of the Royal Statistical Society-B*, 39:1–22, 1977.

[39] D.G.T. Denison, B.K. Mallick, and A.F.M. Smith. A Bayesian CART algorithm. *Biometrika*, 85:363–378, 1998.

[40] L. Devroye, L. Gyorfi, and G. Lugosi. *A Probability Theory of Pattern Recognition*. Springer, New York, 1996.

[41] P.J. Diggle, K.Y. Liang, and S.L. Zeger. *Analysis of Longitudinal Data*. Oxford Science Publications, Oxford, 1991.

[42] B. Efron. Estimating the error rate of a prediction rule: Improvement on cross-validation. *Journal of the American Statistical Association*, 78:316–331, 1983.

[43] R.C. Elston and J. Stewart. A general model for the genetic analysis of pedigree data. *Human Heredity*, 21:523–542, 1971.

[44] B.G. Ferris, F.E. Speizer, J.D. Spengler, D.W. Dockery, Y.M.M. Bishop, M. Wolfson, and C. Humble. Effects of sulfur oxides and respirable particles on human health. *American Review of Respiratory Disease*, 120:767–779, 1979.

[45] G.M. Fitzmaurice and N.M. Laird. A likelihood-based method for analysing longitudinal binary responses. *Biometrika*, 80:141–151, 1993.

[46] G.M. Fitzmaurice and N.M. Laird. Regression models for a bivariate discrete and continuous outcome with clustering. *Journal of the American Statistical Association*, 90:845–852, 1995.

[47] G.M. Fitzmaurice, N.M. Laird, and A.G. Rotnitzky. Regression models for discrete longitudinal responses. *Statistical Science*, 8:284–299, 1993.

[48] T.R. Fleming and D.P. Harrington. *Counting processes and survival analysis*. Wiley, New York, 1991.

[49] J.H. Friedman. A recursive partitioning decision rule for nonparametric classification. *IEEE Trans. Computers*, C-26:404–407, 1977.

[50] J.H. Friedman. Multivariate adpative regression splines. *Annals of Statistics*, 19:1–141, 1991.

[51] J.H. Friedman and B.W. Silverman. Flexible parsimonious smoothing and additive modeling. *Technometrics*, 31:3–21, 1989.

[52] A.M. Garber, R.A. Olshen, H.P. Zhang, and E.S. Venkatraman. Predicting high-risk cholesterol levels. *International Statistical Review*, 62:203–228, 1994.

[53] A. Gersho and R.M. Gray. *Vector Quantization and Signal Compression*. Kluwer, Norwell, Massachusetts, 1992.

[54] E. Giovannucci, A. Ascherio, E.B. Rimm, M.J. Stampfer, G.A. Colditz, and W.C. Willett. Intake of carotenoids and retinol in relation to risk of prostate cancer. *Journal of the National Cancer Institute*, 87:1767–1776, 1995.

[55] V.P. Godambe. An optimum property of regular maximum likelihood estimation. *Annals of Mathematical Statistics*, 31:1209–1211, 1960.

[56] L. Goldman, F. Cook, P. Johnson, D. Brand, G. Rouan, and T. Lee. Prediction of the need for intensive care in patients who come to emergency departments with acute chest pain. *The New England Journal of Medicine*, 334:1498–504, 1996.

[57] L. Goldman, M. Weinberg, R.A. Olshen, F. Cook, R. Sargent, et al. A computer protocol to predict myocardial infarction in emergency department patients with chest pain. *The New England Journal of Medicine*, 307:588–597, 1982.

[58] L. Gordon and R.A. Olshen. Asymptotically efficient solutions to the classification problem. *Annals of Statistics*, 6:515–533, 1978.

[59] L. Gordon and R.A. Olshen. Consistent nonparametric regression from recursive partitioning schemes. *J. Multivariate Analysis*, 10:611–627, 1980.

[60] L. Gordon and R.A. Olshen. Almost surely consistent nonparametric regression from recursive partitioning schemes. *J. Multivariate Analysis*, 15:147–163, 1984.

[61] L. Gordon and R.A. Olshen. Tree-structured survival analysis. *Cancer Treatment Reports*, 69:1065–1069, 1985.

References

[62] P.M. Grambsch and T.M. Therneau. Proportional hazards tests and diagnostics based on weighted residuals. *Biometrika*, 81:515–526, 1994.

[63] J.A. Hanley. Receiver operating characteristic (ROC) methodology: the state of the art. *Clinical Reviews in Diagnostic Imaging*, 29:307–335, 1989.

[64] J.D. Hart and T.E. Wehrly. Kernel regression estimation using repeated measurements data. *Journal of the American Statistical Association*, 81:1080–1088, 1986.

[65] T. Hastie. Comments on Flexible parsimonious smoothing and additive modeling. *Technometrics*, 31:23–29, 1989.

[66] T.J. Hastie and R.J. Tibshirani. *Generalized additive models*. Chapman and Hall, London, 1990.

[67] E.G. Henrichon and K.S. Fu. A nonparametric partitioning procedure for pattern classification. *IEEE Trans. Computers*, C-18:614–624, 1969.

[68] D. Hinkley. Inference in two-phase regression. *Journal of the American Statistical Association*, 66:736–743, 1971.

[69] M. Hollander and F. Proschan. Testing to determine the underlying distribution using randomly censored data. *Biometrics*, 35:393–401, 1979.

[70] P. Huber. *Robust statistics*. John Wiley & Sons, New York, 1981.

[71] O. Intrator and C. Kooperberg. Trees and splines in survival analysis. *Statistical Methods in Medical Research*, 4:237–262, 1995.

[72] J. Kalbfleish and R.L. Prentice. Marginal likelihoods based on Cox's regression and life model. *Biometrika*, 60:267–278, 1973.

[73] J. Kalbfleish and R.L. Prentice. *The Statistical Analysis of Failure Time Data*. Wiley, New York, 1980.

[74] E.L. Kaplan and P. Meier. Nonparametric estimation from incomplete observations. *Journal of the American Statistical Association*, 53:457–481, 1958.

[75] D.G. Kleinbaum, L.L. Kupper, and K.E. Muller. *Applied Regression Analysis and Other Multivariable Methods*. Duxbury Press, Belmont, California, 1988.

[76] L.W. Kwak, J. Halpern, R.A. Olshen, and S.J. Horning. Prognostic significance of actual dose intensity in diffuse large-cell lymphoma: results of a tree-structured survival analysis. *Journal of Clinical Oncology*, 8:963–977, 1990.

[77] N.M. Laird and J.H. Ware. Random-effects models for longitudinal data. *Biometrics*, 38:963–974, 1982.

[78] M. LeBlanc and J. Crowley. Relative risk trees for censored survival data. *Biometrics*, 48:411–425, 1992.

[79] M. LeBlanc and J. Crowley. Survival trees by goodness-of-split. *Journal of the American Statistical Association*, 88:457–467, 1993.

[80] M. LeBlanc and J. Crowley. A review of tree-based prognostic models. In *Recent Advances in Clinical Trial Design and Analysis*, pages 113–124, P.F. Thall, ed. Kluwer, New York, 1995.

[81] E.T. Lee. *Statistical Methods for Survival Data Analysis*. Wiley, New York, 1992.

[82] D.E. Levy, J.J. Caronna, B.H. Singer, et al. Predicting outcome from hypoxic-ischemic coma. *Journal of the American Medical Association*, 253:1420–1426, 1985.

[83] K.Y. Liang and S.L. Zeger. Longitudinal data analysis using generalized linear models. *Biometrika*, 73:13–22, 1986.

[84] K.Y. Liang, S.L. Zeger, and B. Qaqish. Multivariate regression analyses for categorical data. *Journal of the Royal Statistical Society-B*, 54:3–24, 1992.

[85] W.Y. Loh and N. Vanichsetakul. Tree-structured classification via generalized discriminant analysis. *Journal of the American Statistical Association*, 83:715–725, 1988.

[86] W.L. Long, J.L. Griffith, H.P. Selker, and R.B. D'Agostino. A comparison of logistic regression to decision tree induction in a medical domain. *Computers and Biomedical Research*, 26:74–97, 1993.

[87] G. Lugosi and A.B. Nobel. Consistency of data-driven histogram methods for density estimation and classification. *Annals of Statistics*, 24:687–706, 1996.

[88] N. Mantel and W. Haenszel. Statistical aspects of the analysis of data from retrospective studies of disease. *Journal of the National Cancer Institute*, 22:719–48, 1959.

[89] K.M. McConnochie, K.J. Roghmann, and J. Pasternack. Developing prediction rules and evaluating observing patterns using categorical clinical markers: Two complementary procedures. *Medical Decision Making*, 13:30–42, 1993.

[90] P. McCullagh and J.A. Nelder. *Generalized Linear Models*. Chapman and Hall, London, 1989.

[91] C.A. McGilchrist and B.R. Cullis. REML estimation for repeated measures analysis. *Journal of Statistical Computation and Simulation*, 38:151–163, 1991.

[92] G.J. McLachlan and T. Krishnan. *The EM Algorithm and Extensions*. John Wiley & Sons, New York, 1997.

[93] R. Messenger and L. Mandell. A modal search technique for predictive nominal scale multivariate analysis. *Journal of the American Statistical Association*, 67:768–772, 1972.

[94] O.S. Miettinen. Stratification by a multivariate confounder score. *American Journal of Epidemiology*, 104:609–620, 1976.

[95] R.G. Miller. Least squares regression with censored data. *Biometrika*, 63:449–464, 1976.

[96] R.G. Miller. *Survival Analysis*. Wiley, New York, 1981.

[97] R.G. Miller. What price Kaplan–Meier? *Biometrics*, 39:1077–1081, 1983.

[98] P.K. Mills, W.L. Beeson, R.L. Phillips, and G.E. Fraser. Bladder cancer in a low risk population: results from the Adventist Health Study. *American Journal of Epidemiology*, 133:230–239, 1991.

[99] J.N. Morgan and R.C. Messenger *THAID: a sequential search program for the analysis of nominal scale dependent variables*. Institute for Social Research, University of Michigan, Ann Arbor, 1973.

[100] J.N. Morgan and J.A. Sonquist. Problems in the analysis of survey data, and a proposal. *Journal of the American Statistical Association*, 58:415–434, 1963.

[101] A.R. Moss, P. Bcchetti, D. Osmond, W. Krampf, R.E. Chaisson, D. Stites, J. Wilber, J.-P. Allain, and J. Carlson. Seropositive for HIV and the development of AIDS: Three-year follow-up of the San Francisco General Hospital Cohort. *British Medical Journal*, 298:745–750, 1988.

[102] R.A. Moyeed and P.J. Diggle. Rates of convergence in semiparametric modelling of longitudinal data. *Australian Journal of Statistics*, 36:75–93, 1994.

[103] W. Nelson. On estimating the distribution of a random vector when only the coordinate is observable. *Technometrics*, 12:923–924, 1969.

[104] W. Nelson. Theory and applications of hazard plotting for censored failure data. *Technometrics*, 14:945–966, 1972.

[105] A.B. Nobel. Histogram regression estimation using data-dependent partitions. *Annals of Statistics*, 24:1084–1105, 1996.

[106] A.B. Nobel and R.A. Olshen. Termination and continuity of greedy growing for tree structured vector quantizers. *IEEE Transactions on Information Theory*, 42:191–206, 1996.

[107] H.D. Patterson and R. Thompson. Recovery of inter-block information when block sizes are unequal. *Biometrika*, 58:545–554, 1971.

[108] R. Peto. Experimental survival curves for interval-censored data. *Applied Statistics*, 22:86–91, 1973.

[109] R. Peto and J. Peto. Asymptotically efficient rank invariant test procedures (with discussion). *Journal of the Royal Statistical Society-A*, 135:185–206, 1972.

[110] G. Poggi and R.A. Olshen. Pruned tree-structured vector quantization of medical images with segmentation and improved prediction. *IEEE Transactions on Image Processing*, 4:734–741, 1995.

[111] D.R. Ragland, R.J. Brand, et al. Coronary heart disease mortality in the western collaborative group study: Follow-up experience of 22 years. *American Journal of Epidemiology*, 127:462–475, 1988.

[112] E.G. Raymond, N. Tafari, J.F. Troendle, and J.D. Clemens. Development of a practical screening tool to identify preterm, low-birthweight neonates in Ethiopia. *Lancet*, 344:520–523, 1994.

[113] J.A. Rice and B.W. Silverman. Estimating the mean and covariance structure nonparametrically when the data are curves. *Journal of the Royal Statistical Society-B*, 53:233–243, 1991.

[114] A.M. Richardson and A.H. Welsh. Asymptotic properties of restricted maximum likelihood (REML) estimates for hierarchical mixed linear models. *The Australian Journal of Statistics*, 36:31–43, 1994.

[115] R.M. Royall. Model robust inference using maximum likelihood estimators. *International Statistical Review*, 54:221–226, 1986.

[116] I.R. Savage. Contributions to the theory of rank order statistics—the two sample case. *Annals of Mathematical Statistics*, 27:590–615, 1956.

[117] J. Scourfield, D.E. Stevens, and K.R. Merikangas. Substance abuse, comorbidity, and sensation seeking: gender difference. *Comprehensive Psychiatry*, 37:384–392, 1996.

[118] M.R. Segal. Regression trees for censored data. *Biometrics*, 44:35–48, 1988.

[119] M.R. Segal. Tree-structured methods for longitudinal data. *Journal of the American Statistical Association*, 87:407–418, 1992.

[120] M.R. Segal. Extending the elements of tree-structured regression. *Statistical Methods in Medical Research*, 4:219–236, 1995.

[121] M.R. Segal and D. Bloch. A comparison of estimated proportional hazards models and regression trees. *Statistics in Medicine*, 8:539–550, 1989.

[122] M.R. Segal and D.A. Bloch. A comparison of estimated proportional hazards models and regression trees. *Statistics in Medicine*, 8:539–550, 1989.

[123] H.P. Selker, J.L. Griffith, S. Patil, W.L. Long, and R.B. D'Agostino. A comparison of performance of mathematical predictive methods for medical diagnosis: Identifying acute cardiac ischemia among emergency department patients. *Journal of Investigative Medicine*, 43:468–476, 1995.

[124] B.W. Silverman. Some aspects of the spline smoothing approach to non-parametric regression curve fitting. *Journal of the Royal Statistical Society-B*, 47:1–21, 1985.

[125] P.L. Smith. Curve fitting and modeling with splines using statistical variable selection techniques. NASA 166034, Langley Research Center, Hampton, VA, 1982.

[126] A. Sommer, J. Katz, and I. Tarwotjo. Increased risk of respiratory disease and diarrhea in children with preexisting mild vitamin A deficiency. *American Journal of Clinical Nutrition*, 40:1090–1095, 1984.

[127] A. Sommer, I. Tarwotjo, G. Hussaini, and D. Susanto. Increased mortality in children with mild vitamin A deficiency. *Lancet*, 2:585–588, 1983.

[128] A. Sommer, J.M. Tielsch, J. Katz, H.A. Quigley, J.D. Gottsch, J.C. Javitt, J.F. Martone, R.M. Royall, K.A. Witt, and S. Ezrine. Racial differences in the cause-specific prevalence of blindness in east Baltimore. *New England Journal of Medicine*, 325:1412–1417, 1991.

[129] StatSci. *S-PLUS: Guide to Statistical and Mathematical Analyis*. MathSoft, Inc., Seattle, 1993.

[130] StatSci. *S-PLUS: Guide to Statistical and Mathematical Analyis*. MathSoft, Inc., Seattle, 1995.

[131] D.M. Stier, J.M. Leventhal, A.T. Berg, L. Johnson, and J. Mezger. Are children born to young mothers at increased risk of maltreatment? *Pediatrics*, 91:642–648, 1993.

[132] N.R. Temkin, R. Holubkov, J.E. Machamer, H.R. Winn, and S.S. Dikmen. Classification and regression trees (CART) for prediction of function at 1 year following head trauma. *Journal of Neurosurgery*, 82:764–771, 1995.

[133] T.M. Therneau, P.M. Grambsch, and T.R. Fleming. Martingale-based residuals for survival models. *Biometrika*, 77:147–160, 1990.

[134] A. Tishler and I. Zang. A new maximum likelihood algorithm for piecewise regression. *Journal of the American Statistical Association*, 76:980–987, 1981.

[135] Y.K. Truong. Nonparametric curve estimation with time series errors. *Journal of Statistical Planning and Inference*, 28:167–183, 1991.

[136] J.H. Ware, D.W. Dockery, A. Spiro, F.E. Speizer, and B.G. Ferris. Passive smoking, gas cooking, and respiratory health of children living in six cities. *American Review of Respiratory Disease*, 129:366–374, 1984.

[137] D.R. Wasserman and J.M. Leventhal. Maltreatment of children born to cocaine-dependent mothers. *American Journal of Diseases of Children*, 147:1324–1328, 1993.

[138] R.J. Young and B.A. Bod. Development of computer-directed methods for the identification of hyperactivated motion using motion patterns developed by rabbit sperm during incubation under capacitation conditions. *Journal of Andrology*, 15:362–377, 1994.

[139] S.L. Zeger and P.J. Diggle. Semiparametric models for longitudinal data with application to CD4 cell numbers in HIV seroconverters. *Biometrics*, 50:689–699, 1994.

References

[140] S.L. Zeger, K.Y. Liang, and P.S. Albert. Models for longitudinal data: A generalized estimating equation approach. *Biometrics*, 44:1049–1060, 1988.

[141] H.P. Zhang. *Confidence Regions in Nonlinear Regression and Geometry*. Ph.D. Dissertation, Department of Statistics, Stanford University, 1991.

[142] H.P. Zhang. Maximal correlation and adaptive splines. *Technometrics*, 36:196–201, 1994.

[143] H.P. Zhang. Splitting criteria in survival trees. In *Statistical Modelling: Proceedings of the 10th International Workshop on Statistical Modelling*, pages 305–314, Innsbruck, Austria, July 1995a. Springer-Verlag.

[144] H.P. Zhang. Classification trees for multiple binary responses. *Journal of the American Statistical Association*, 93:180–193, 1998a.

[145] H.P. Zhang. Comments on Bayesian CART model search. *Journal of the American Statistical Association*, 93:948–950, 1998b.

[146] H.P. Zhang. Analysis of infant growth curves using MASAL. *Biometrics*, to appear, 1999.

[147] H.P. Zhang and M.B. Bracken. Tree-based risk factor analysis of preterm delivery and small-for-gestational-age birth. *American Journal of Epidemiology*, 141:70–78, 1995.

[148] H.P. Zhang and M.B. Bracken. Tree-based, two-stage risk factor analysis for spontaneous abortion. *American Journal of Epidemiology*, 144:989–996, 1996.

[149] H.P. Zhang, J. Crowley, H.C. Sox, and R.A. Olshen. Tree-structured statistical methods. *Encyclopedia of Biostatistics*, 6:4561–4573, 1998.

[150] H.P. Zhang, T. Holford, and M.B. Bracken. A tree-based method of analysis for prospective studies. *Statistics in Medicine*, 15:37–49, 1996.

[151] H.P. Zhang and K.R. Merikangas. Analysis of familial transmission of alcoholism using frailty models. *Unpublished manuscript*, 1999.

[152] L.P. Zhao and R.L. Prentice. Correlated binary regression using a quadratic exponential model. *Biometrika*, 77:642–648, 1990.

Index

1-SE rule, 40

adaptive splines, 6, 105
adaptive splines model, 115, 128–130
additive model, 132
adjusted 2 × 2 table, 48
AIC, 100
allowable splits, 10, 11, 59, 101
    ordinal variables, 10
    continuous, 10
    nominal variables, 11
association, 61
association parameter, 177
autocorrelation, 140
Automatic Interaction Detection, 15
automatic interaction detection (AID), 15

back-fitting algorithm, 143
backward stepwise, 23–25, 91
Bahadur representation, 178
basis function, 105, 116–118, 120, 121, 123, 128, 130
    cubic, 128, 129
basis vector, 120, 121, 129
binary response, 21, 173
    longitudinal, 174, 195
binary tree, 15
binomial distribution, 31
Breslow's estimate, 98

canonical parameters, 176
CART, 1–3
case-control study, 30
censoring, 72
    indicator, 74
    interval, 73
    left, 73
    right, 73
    type I, 72
    type II, 73
    type III, 73
censoring time, 74
classification trees for multiple binary responses (CTMBR), 6, 183
collinearity, 132
competitive split, 54

complexity parameter, 35–44, 119
    threshold, 36
compound symmetry, 147
conditional expectation, 4
conditional probability, 4
cost-complexity, 35, 100, 120, 184
covariance structure, 142
    conditional independence, 141
    Gaussian form, 153
    stationary form, 147
Cox model, 89, 97
cross-validation, 16, 27, 35, 39, 56
    generalized, 119
    localized, 47

delta splitting rule, 32
deviance, 98
dichotomous variable, 4
discriminant analysis, 3
distribution function
    improper, 95

EM algorithm, 168, 183
end-cut preference, 31, 185
entropy, 30
    generalized, 183
    impurity, 12
error
    Bayes, 30
    minimum, 30
    nearest neighbor, 30
estimate
    cross-validation, 40, 48, 49
        standard error, 40
    product-limit, 84
    resubstitution, 26, 34, 48
    test sample, 40
estimating equations
    GEE, 180
    GEE1, 180
    GEE2, 180
    generalized, 180

F-errors, 30
failure rate
    instantaneous, 81
false negative error, 33
false positive error, 33
false positive probability, 26
family founder, 182
fixed-effect, 140
frailty model, 181

Gaussian process, 143, 148
GCV, 119, 132, 134
Gini index, 30, 184
growth curve, 152, 153, 159, 161

hazard
    baseline, 90
    constant, 81, 96
    cumulative, 97
    proportional, 91, 97
hazard function, 81
    cumulative, 82
hazard plotting, 82

impurity, 30, 95
indicator function, 74

Kaplan–Meier curve, 82, 84, 94, 101
kernel estimate, 144
knot, 115–130

learning sample, 9, 99, 185, 189
least squares, 116, 117, 121
likelihood function, 22, 31
    conditional, 89, 90
    full, 81, 97
    partial, 97
linear regression, 4, 105
link function, 180
    logit, 21
log-linear models, 176
log-rank test, 85, 96, 100, 101
longitudinal data, 137, 139, 141–145, 166, 167
longitudinal studies, 137

marginal model, 178

marginal parameters, 178
Markov Chain Monte Carlo, 56
MARS, 1, 105
    backward algorithm, 118
    forward algorithm, 115
MASAL, 144–168
maximal correlation, 125, 127
maximum likelihood, 22
minimum span, 124, 127
misclassification cost, 32–43
    conditional, 34
    unconditional, 34
    unit of, 33
    within-node, 34
misclassification rate, 3
missing data, 24–25, 53, 54
missings together (MT), 53–54
mixed model, 140
mixed-effects model, 140
morbidity, 3
mortality, 3
multinomial distribution, 177

Nelson's estimate, 98
Newton-Raphson method, 22
node, 9
    minimum size, 15
    terminal, 15
    daughter, 9
    homogeneity, 183, 184, 195
    impurity, 10, 29–32, 184
    internal, 9
    parent, 9
    partition, 9
    root, 9, 59
    terminal, 9
nonparametric model, 144
normal density, 4

odds, 22
odds ratio, 22, 25, 177
    adjusted, 22, 67
optimal subtree, 36, 39
    nested, 39
outcome, 4

pairwise correlation, 186
pedigree, 175
piecewise linear function, 105, 113
piecewise polynomials, 105
polytomous responses, 195
prediction rule, 4
predictor, 4
    nominal, 23
preterm delivery, 3, 7
prevalence rate, 30
prior, 30
probability plotting, 82
proportional hazard model, 89
prospective studies, 30
pruning, 15
    alternative procedures, 43
    bottom-up, 100
pruning rules, 100

quadratic exponential model, 176
quasi-score function, 181

random variable, 4
random-effect, 140
receiver operating characteristic, 25
    ROC curves, 25, 49, 52
recursive partitioning, 1–6, 10, 14–32, 54, 59, 93
regression, 1
    proportional hazard, 1
    linear, 1, 143
    logistic, 1, 3–23, 63
    nonparametric, 1
    parametric, 1
regression trees, 105, 167–169
regressive logistic models, 181
relative risk, 44
    adjusted, 63
    confidence interval, 49
    crude, 63
REML, 145
risk set, 90
RTREE, 16

SAS, 22

semiparametric model, 143
sensitivity, 26
specificity, 26
spline model, 105
split
    goodness of, 11–31, 58, 59
    twoing rule, 31
spontaneous abortion, 61
stopping rules, 15
subadditivity, 184
subtree, 32, 35
surrogate splits , 53–55
survival function, 79, 81, 97
    exponential, 82
survival time, 71, 72
    censored, 72
survival trees, 6
swapping, 19

test sample, 35, 39
THAID, 32
time trend, 144
tree
    repair, 43
    stability, 55
true positive probability, 26
truncated function, 112, 113, 117, 120, 128

uniform correlation, 147

validation sample, 35, 189
variables
    dummy, 23, 25, 50, 108, 152, 159, 161, 195, 196
    nominal, 11, 59
variogram, 163

Wasserstein metrics, 94
Western Collaborative Group Study, 74, 79

Yale Pregnancy Outcome Study, 7, 9, 40, 61